Contents

Abbreviations

AHA	area health authority
BMA	British Medical Association
CCS	(MacMillan) continuing care service
CHC	community health council
DHA	district health authority
DHSS	Department of Health and Social Security
FNEHAD	Fédération Nationale des Etablissements d'Hospitalisation à Domicile (France)
FPC	family practitioner committee
GP	general practitioner
HAD	*hospitalisation à domicile* (France)
HAH	hospital at home
HSA	hospital savings association
LASSD	local authority social services department
MOH	Ministry of Health; Medical Officer of Health
NHS	National Health Service
NHI	national health insurance
NSCR	National Society for Cancer Relief
UK	United Kingdom

Acknowledgements

To acknowledge everyone who has helped me either directly or indirectly to formulate the ideas contained in this book would be impossible. Their influence extends to a time long before I first set pen to paper. Some, however, must be singled out for special mention:

Friends, colleagues and patients of Barnet General Hospital, alongside whom I worked for many years through a series of health reorganisations.

The British Council, whose fellowship award in 1972 enabled the first of my numerous visits to study *hospitalisation à domicile* (HAD) in France; the Nuffield Foundation which, in 1977, enabled a joint study visit to various HAD schemes together with Stephen Cang of the Health Services Organisation Research Unit, Brunel University; the Sainsbury Family Charitable Trusts, whose generous grant made possible the first 'hospital at home' experiment under the NHS.

The pioneers and personnel of the Paris, Bayonne, Bordeaux and Grenoble HAD schemes in France, who were unstinting in the time and trouble they took to describe their aims and organisations; nurses and social workers of these schemes, with whom I visited many patients; pioneers and personnel of hospital-based home care schemes in Adelaide and Melbourne (Australia) and Auckland (New Zealand) who kindly wrote to me describing their experiences.

The many people throughout the UK who wrote to me, following publication in the early 1970s of articles on the French HAD experience, urging practical action towards the setting up of similar services under the NHS, including health administrators, doctors and nurses, university staff, members of community health councils and other organisations of patient concern.

Members and staff of the Cambridgeshire Area Health Authority (Teaching), in particular of the Peterborough District, with whom I shared some both stressful and immensely rewarding times; members of the Peterborough Hospital at Home scheme's steering group; the first patients of the Peterborough Hospital at Home scheme, whose testimony of the benefits of HAH left no doubt in the mind as to the need throughout the NHS for realistic alternatives to general hospital admission.

Finally, on a personal note, I should like to thank Joyce Meadows and Shirley Johnston for their painstaking help in typing successive drafts of this book, Ruth Richardson for her help and guidance in its literary expression, and Arthur and Richard Clarke for their suggestions, criticisms and morale-boosting support through many difficult times.

No person other than myself bears any responsibility for the validity of the historical material contained in this book, nor for its interpretation.

Barnet, Herts, 1984   FC

Introduction

Hospital at Home is a title borrowed from '*hospitalisation à domicile*', the name of hospital-based schemes designed to provide options of home care for certain traditionally hospitalised patients in France. These schemes guarantee to the latter predetermined levels and varieties of care, including specialist care, in parallel with those provided in general hospitals. Their 'beds' are included in the official bed complements of the regional hospital authorities responsible for them.

The British system of medicine, whereby general practitioners (GPs) must refer cases to hospitals before patients can receive specialist care, has been with us for so long that it is now difficult to envisage any other. It entails organisational separation between hospital and community sectors of the National Health Service (NHS). Measures taken by the NHS to bring these sectors together operationally have not by and large reached the medical profession because GPs and specialists are deeply resistant to integrated ways of working, other than on an informal basis.

Reasons for divisions in British medicine can be traced far back in history. Many generations of specialists have fought against incursion into hospital medicine by their GP colleagues, while the latter have retaliated by defending their work amongst the sick outside hospitals from incursion by specialists. This has led to a two-tier system in medicine, whereby 'primary' care takes place in the community and 'secondary' provision is confined to hospitals. Of course, many patients suffering major illnesses are looked after in their own homes. But it is assumed that any specialist treatment they might need can be adequately met through their hospital out-patient attendances; while their basic support is the responsibility of their families, possibly helped by local authority social services departments.

As doctors, nurses and health administrators are well aware, this concept does not fit well with reality. Many patients at home suffer unnecessarily and are denied recovery prospects because they do not have access to specialist treatment and hospital-held resources. Equally, many hospitalised patients could be more effectively cared for at home, given the availability there of specialist treatment and levels, varieties and patterns of care similar to those traditionally available to them only in hospitals.

This irrational state of affairs has persisted because health authorities here are empowered only to provide 'items' of medical and nursing care in the community. The nature of these items is determined by GPs, who may or may not be willing and able to identify and act upon the specialist and basic support needs of their patients. Since GPs are independently contracted to the NHS, and are hence not accountable to district health authorities, there are no means by which the latter can monitor or regulate their work. The level and quality of nursing services available to patients in their own homes depends largely on individual GP qualities, since, by and large, community nurses and health visitors work through a system of GP attachments.

Most families look after their sick members without external help. Where GPs observe a need for this it is usually met in a piecemeal, loosely monitored way, fluctuating according to whether or not family breakdown appears imminent. If this actually occurs, emergency hospital admissions can be arranged.

Ideally, every patient for whom hospital admission is not crucial for medical reasons should have the opportunity to be cared for in the environment of home and family, and should be provided with external basic support where this is lacking and with specialist skills and resources where the need for these is medically indicated. Some patients, however, must be admitted to hospital because their treatments involve the use of equipment and/or skills in such short supply that they must be centred where the greatest possible number of patients can benefit from them. Others must be admitted because home and family environment cannot be modified to meet their requirements. Between these extremes, many patients have no option but to enter hospital whenever their GPs are unwilling or unable to attend them at home. Only patients who can afford to pay privately for requisite medical (including specialist), nursing and domestic help are able to choose their environments of treatment.

More home care of the sick in Britain than at present might be possible through a straight transfer of NHS resources from hospital to community health services. But the latter do not have the powers or organisation necessary to ensure their effective and economic use. Furthermore, they lack authority to reach explicit agreement with families of the sick, necessary to co-ordinate contributions of the latter with those of a statutory nature.

An undercurrent of discontent about alleged inequable distribution of health resources between hospital and community sectors has afflicted the NHS since its creation. This has never been permitted to surface in ways enabling objective consideration of optimum consumer requirements. Community health councils set up to help determine these are inhibited by the fact that GP services fall outside their terms of reference. If they *could* be determined, health authorities would not be able to act on findings in favour of high levels and wide varieties of community provision, because they do not hold the powers necessary for their close monitoring and control.

There is now stalemate in the NHS between hospital/ community and specialist/GP services. We know that hospital beds are blocked by patients who do not essentially require them, while patients who do are placed on long waiting lists. We know that many patients suffer ill effects from hospital admissions when, given the availability of special facilities, they could be better looked after at home. We know that probably most GPs would like to have access to hospital beds and that most hospital specialists would like to offer options of home care for certain of their patients. Yet, neither health authorities nor Government appear capable of action cutting across divisions in medicine which would enable specialists and GPs to treat their patients, alternatively, at home or in hospital, according to the aspirations of the patient.

Hospital at Home conveys a concept new to British medicine. It has been written in a belief that patients suffering major illness in their own homes require an approach to their needs similar to that which applies to hospitalised patients. Since this is currently impossible under the NHS, I have looked overseas in the hope of discovering whether the same applies to all health systems. I have found that doctors nearly everywhere are divided into two main classes of generalist and specialist; but in Britain the division is wider and more rigid than in most countries, due to the way in which medical care is organised here. Elsewhere, divisions are not essentially collinear with those of community and hospital. This has provided scope in certain overseas countries for experiment in comprehensive home care for the dependent sick of a kind which is currently not feasible here.

In France many '*hospitalisation à domicile*' (HAD) schemes have now passed their experimental stages to become permanent features of regional hospital provision. They rely for their budgets on annual agreements reached between the particular hospital authorities sponsoring them and the. 'Securité Sociale' (the regionally organised state insurance body which reimburses patients at rates between 80 per cent and 100 per cent of hospital expenses). Through their national federation these schemes between them adopt similar structures, operational patterns and codes of practice. Fundamental to these is the concept that patients accepted by them must first have been given options between general hospital and HAD admission: that these must take into account the wishes of family members directly involved in the event of an option in favour of HAD. Certain conditions have to be met before the option can be offered: patients must be considered by their doctors to require levels and varieties of care normally indicating need for general hospital admission; a doctor must signify willingness to accept clinical responsibility for the arrangement in each case. Otherwise, the extent to which these schemes might be developed depends on their financial viability and the availability of skills and personnel which, it might be claimed, could be more economically deployed in treating patients *en masse* in hospitals.

Great lay and professional interest in the French experience was demonstrated in Britain in response to articles on the subject published during the early 1970s (see chapters 4 and 5). This led to pressure for similar experiments under the NHS. The opportunity arose when a charitable trust offered a generous grant to a health authority willing to undertake a three-year project based on the French experience. There were numerous contenders for the grant, which was finally awarded to the Peterborough Health District of the Cambridgeshire Area Health Authority (Teaching), whose Hospital at Home three-year pilot scheme was launched in 1978 (see chapter 7)

Numerous other home care pilot schemes, often aimed at reducing pressure on hospital beds, have been set up in the UK over the past two decades. Most have been enabled by joint health–social services funding. Some, administered by local authority social services departments, cater for persons no longer in need of major treatments, but nevertheless too disabled and infirm to cope at home with the help of traditional community services. Others cater for patients requiring 'items' of treatment – for example, dressings and the removal of stitches – which, in the absence of the schemes, would involve the patient's continued stay in hospital. These are administered by community nursing services in liaison with hospital units.

Programmes of continuing hospital/community care for particular groups of patients – for example, the paediatric, the geriatric and the terminally ill – have been in operation in some parts of the UK for many years: some at the initiative of hospital units; some inspired by religious foundations and supported, at least in part, by charity. Their prime interest is not to conserve hospital beds but rather, as far as is possible, to meet patient and family aspirations. Excellent as they often are, they cannot meet criteria considered crucial (in this volume) to adequate patient and family protection because they are tied to divided medical, health and social services, described above. No single administration, therefore, can be designated responsible for assuring overall case requirements.

I have devoted the early pages of this book to a brief study of the growth of British medicine. This has been necessary to enable understanding of the far-reaching fundamental implications of HAH for doctors (GPs and specialists), other health professionals and administrators, social workers and, above all, patients and their families. Passing reference to known home care initiatives in various overseas countries indicates the extent of global interest in the search for alternatives to hospital admission. I have discussed in detail the French experience because it demonstrates in tangible ways the crucial importance of sound administration and organisation in domiciliary provision for patients suffering major illness and incapacity.

The extent and variety of health and local authority, as well as individual and group voluntary, effort aimed at meeting the existing shortfall in NHS provision for home care can be judged from examples included in chapter 6. First-hand experience of HAH as practised at Peterborough, described in chapter 7, gives readers an idea of the extent of GP and community nursing resistance to experiment in organisationally merged community and hospital services. On the part of hospital staff it suggests wide interest in such an experiment, but scepticism about prospects of breaking down resistance to their participation in home care on the community side. The Peterborough experiment leaves us in no doubt about the crucial need for a category of health workers new to the NHS, here referred to as patients' aides, who would provide, under nursing management, all the basic support which patients' families are unable themselves to provide.

In the final chapters of this book I have attempted to predict advantages which would accrue to health professionals in this country through a merging of hospital and GP services such as I have envisaged in this volume: NHS administrators, hospital clinicians, nurses, paramedical and social workers, community workers and those responsible for decision-making in social services would all, I believe, thereby be enabled to plan their work (in directions of both prevention and cure) towards the optimum economic, effective and humane advantage of those whom they serve and to their own professional gain. My findings are potentially of great relevance to a wide spectrum of degrees and training courses, also to health unions and their members.

Lay organisations such as community health councils, community action groups, special patient interest and other voluntary bodies – indeed, all who come into contact with the sick – will find in ideas expressed in this book ways in which those whom they seek to help might gain from integrated hospital and GP services advantages presently denied to them as a result of their division.

I Pre-twentieth-century health provision in Britain: an introductory sketch

Unnecessary hospital admissions have long been a subject of concern to doctors and administrators; a concern which centres mainly on cost and the use of hospital beds in short supply. But there is also growing concern amongst all sections of society about the harm which may be caused by removal to hospital at times when we are particularly vulnerable to pressures from which home and family traditionally protect us. At such times we may be incapable of action to avoid such removal, so it is a relief to know that doctors have the responsibility of deciding when it should take place.

If doctors were always motivated and in a position to act in the best interests of their patients, in the full knowledge of what those interests might be, this arrangement might provide the happiest feasible solution to problems of illness for both patient and doctor. Unhappily this is not the case. Despite the fact that doctors are as liable to failings of human motivation as are members of other professional groups, the medical profession has over the years carved for itself patterns of health care which leave the sick little alternative but to place themselves in the hands of the particular doctor with whom they happen to be registered.

Generations of GPs have chosen or been obliged to hospitalise their patients in order that the latter might receive specialist attention, and/or be fully cared for whilst undergoing treatment. Many of those patients might have been more effectively nursed at home, given the availability there of specialist treatment adequate basic care. Once in hospital many hav disastrous consequences, not of their original illn

7

those of being institutionalised, regimented and subjected to
sometimes excessive examination and medication.

The NHS reflects both the best and worst features of
traditional medicine, to which have been harnessed achievements of modern science and technology. But, with increasing
evidence that use of the latter is prone to create as well as resolve
illness, doctors now have an obligation to exercise greater caution
than they may have done in the past to avoid exposing their
patients to unecessary dangers. If the medical profession accepts
that hospitals are potentially dangerous environments for the
sick, it is faced with an obligation to press, where possible, for
alternatives in environments which do not hold the same
dangers. Since some of these dangers apply to all patients treated
in groups, it follows that, wherever possible, these environments
should be their own homes.

We need to know something of the past history of patient services
because some present-day medical practices are rooted in the past; as
too are the reasons why many more patients than at present cannot
be adequately treated and cared for in their own homes.

Hospitals and doctors of the past

The broad pattern of modern health provision in the Western
democracies, including Britain, has been largely set in the past by
medical practice and organisation based on hospitals. Thus it is
to the latter that we must first look to determine how it came
about that patients' homes have come to be regarded as
unsuitable places for the treatment of major illness.

In the Middle Ages the common people relied mainly on the
advice of wise women of varying competence in their neighbourhoods for their medication; if, indeed, they took any at all. Prior
to the establishment of independent hospital schools in the
twelfth century, the sick amongst the destitute poor, sheltered in
monasteries and convents, were attended by priest-physicians
keen to learn about the human body, whereby to advise and treat
their fee-paying clientele among the wealthy. Accordingly, these
physicians came to regard the sick in two separate lights: those
who had no rights of any kind and who were therefore freely

available to them for whatever purpose they might wish, and those who were entitled by reason of payment to dictate their own conditions of patronage. The sick, in return, regarded their doctors either with deference, grateful for medical attention on any terms, or as social inferiors or equals.

When Henry VIII ordered the dissolution of the monasteries in the mid-sixteenth century, he avoided public outcry by promising Parliament he would ensure that the sick and poor should not suffer as a result. This made way for the passing of the Elizabethan Poor Law Act of 1601, requiring local authorities to provide for the necessary relief of the lame, impotent, old, blind and such others as were unable to work. Workhouse provision which followed was totally unsuited to the needs of the sick. Until the great hospital movement of the nineteenth century, the only hospital accommodation open to commoners was that provided by five royal or chartered hospitals petitioned for by dignitaries of the City of London and in use by the end of the sixteenth century.[1]

During the Middle Ages physicians were ignorant of human anatomy and fought shy of laying hands on patients, relying on long dissertations about their conditions to impress them, the giving of drugs and regulation of diet. There were several ranks of surgeons, ranging from those of barbers, who performed acts such as blood-letting, to the higher surgeons who aspired to the social standing of physicians. This they could hardly expect as their practices were painful, messy and dangerous.[2] Apothecaries, of whom records date from pre-Christian times, worked amongst the lower classes of society not of interest to the physicians and higher surgeons. They engaged mainly in the dispensing of drugs, competing for custom with the wise women who frequently attended the sick free of charge or for very little reward. Apothecaries were beneath the regard of physicians and, although they had no licence to practise, their activities did not at first concern the physicians, who had no wish to extend their own practices amongst a clientele potentially incapable of meeting high fees. The presence of apothecaries in hospitals was, however, indispensable to physicians, who required their assistance in carrying out treatments prescribed by themselves. In addition to the making-up and dispensing of medicines, these apothecaries were required to perform or supervise bleeding, cuppings and blisterings, to supervise bathings, to maintain machines (where they existed) and to look after surgical instruments. They also acted as secretaries to the physicians. Above all, they were required to be available in hospitals at all times.

Such was the difference in status between physicians and surgeons of the Middle Ages that, while the Royal College of Physicians was established in 1518, surgeons did not gain similar recognition until the late eighteenth century. As both physicians and higher surgeons came to appreciate their need for practices amongst the lower classes, they found that they could do this only by bringing patients of the latter to their hospitals. For one thing, they were afraid of entering the homes of the poor; for another, apothecaries were determined to establish for themselves exclusive rights of practice outside hospitals in fields traditionally their own. From the late seventeenth century onwards, jealous guarding of territories changed to open warfare between respective professional bodies (apothecaries having broken away from their fellow 'Mystery of Grocers' in 1617 and established rights to treat the sick in their own homes during the plague of 1665, when many physicians fled from town to country with their wealthy clients[3]).

Measures and counter-measures between apothecaries and physicians, which followed throughout the eighteenth century, were designed in part to provide for the exclusion of charlatans and quacks from medical practice altogether; in part to reinforce status divisions. At the time the social position of all doctors had declined to an extraordinary extent, as also had their incomes. They felt they had a struggle for survival on their hands. No-one seemed quite sure who was and who was not a qualified practitioner. The chaos was not resolved until 1858, when the General Council of Medical Education and Registration (GMC) was created. This required all practising doctors to register, the GMC confirming the status of apothecaries as *bona fide* doctors but providing for the Royal Colleges of Physicians and Surgeons to confer on selected doctors specialist qualification.

Powerful interests of the Royal Colleges ensured the exclusion of apothecaries (in their roles as doctors) from hospitals. GPs, registered with the GMC, were now, however, in a position to establish positions for themselves outside hospitals which could not be usurped by specialists.[4]

Alongside reforms specific to medicine, there was now growing awareness among the upper classes that provision of certain universally available health and sanitation facilities was as crucial to their own health interests as to those of commoners. The industrial revolution had caused drastic deterioration in the living conditions of the latter. Enclosures had prevented them from growing their own food. Resulting changes in methods of agriculture had led to unemployment and migration to towns in search of work. This in turn led to expansion in population and industry, resulting in widespread disease. Whereas the rich had previously been hedged against the effects of this, they were now unable to avoid contact with the labouring classes. When the cholera epidemic of 1831 spread to their ranks, through their contact with servants and factory employees, they began to take an interest in preventive measures and the provision of isolation and treatment facilities suitable, if necessary, for their own use. Hence the first fever hospitals represented a vast improvement on any previous local government hospital provision.

The passing of the Metropolitan Poor Law Act of 1867 was a major step in English social history. It represented the first explicit acknowledgement that it was the duty of the state to provide hospitals for the poor (as distinct from paupers): but it also confirmed local authorities' responsibilities to make hospital (including fever hospital) accommodation available where necessary to all sick persons living within their catchment areas. Although the Act was specific to London, its influence spread rapidly throughout the country. It was followed by massive growth of local authority hospitals of all kinds, no longer tainted with the stigma of Poor Law. By now even the Central Poor Law Board required its institutions to provide 'all reasonable and proper appliances for the treatment of disease of every kind',[5] decreeing that henceforth sick ward fittings were to be of the sort usually provided in the wards of general hospitals. By 1888 every London infirmary had its own medical superintendent, aided by a full-time medical officer, and, for the first time, inmates were referred to as 'patients' not 'paupers'.[6]

The function of these new infirmaries was crystallised by the change from lay to medical administration. Medical superintendents were strongly influenced by standards of teaching hospitals, where all had trained and many had held appointments. Qualified nurses trained in teaching hospitals joined forces with these medical superintendents, taking up posts as matrons in place of often unqualified nurses who might well be the wives of workhouse masters. Schools of nursing were set up in some local authority hospitals. Although these schools could not hope to attract recruits of similar calibre to the well educated and socially elite women to be found in the famous teaching hospitals, they at least assured basic minimum nursing practices and provided working-class women, for the most part dedicated to the care of the sick, with opportunities for formal qualification.

Meanwhile, outside hospitals, changes of equally crucial significance to the care of the sick were taking place. Working men's clubs, employers' associations and friendly societies, interested in insurance against sickness, required the services of doctors for sick members for whom hospital admission was not necessary or feasible. GPs unable to secure their livings through private practice were obliged to accept contracts offered by such organisations. These GPs found it highly distasteful to work under contract to associations of tradesmen, or, worse, their employees. Furthermore, terms of contract were frequently of a kind which made it impossible for them to satisfy their own senses of professional commitment. For example, one club surgery in Birmingham allowed only one minute per patient of consultation time.[7]

Although GPs resented having to comply with regulations of their panel work, they recognised the benefits to themselves of its spread to a working population now interested in medical attention from qualified doctors. Where insurance did not cover a particular treatment, a patient might now find the means to pay for it privately; while workers might be encouraged to pay for medical attention to members of their families not covered by insurance.

Nursing history

Throughout its history the medical profession has always largely determined patterns of virtually all services connected with the care of the sick. Nursing, however, often plays the major part in patient recovery and comfort.

Hospitals invariably employ nurses. The nursing needs of their patients are assessed and assured by nurse-managers. Sick persons at home (and some are more ill than many hospitalised patients) must rely on support from families, friends and neighbours. GPs can be relied upon to enlist the help of paid nurses in clinical treatments (injections, dressings, for example). But they vary from one to the other in their interests in, and capacities to identify, nursing needs in connection with, for example, incontinence, sick-room hygiene and general patient care.

Regardless of resource levels, community nursing services are not and never have been organisationally capable of ensuring satisfaction of the needs of all home-bound patients; relying as they do on GP prescriptions and on administrations covering the whole field of community health ranging from prevention of illness to terminal care.

To understand why so many patients have to be hospitalised when, given adequate nursing, they might have been more successfully treated at home, we need to know something of the history of nursing.

Organised nurse training first took place in convents and monasteries, some of which extended their work to local communities. To the religious dedication of the nurses involved were added disciplines learned in the field hospitals of the Crusades, notably under orders such as those of St John and the Knights of Malta.[8] Apart from on the battlefields, few doctors of medieval times were attached to hospitals – they were called in when nurses considered it necessary and were reimbursed for their services. Thus, while medicine advanced to become a very lucrative profession, nursing remained a calling of dedication, sometimes tempered with military-style discipline, until it became tainted with degradations connected with the Poor Law.[9]

With the rise of Protestantism, many monastic institutions were closed and religious orders destroyed. In both Catholic and Protestant countries most male nurses were removed from their posts, setting the future of nursing as a career for women. Nurses who had worked in religious orders were obliged to take up ill-paid posts in the new Poor Law workhouses, to be assisted by local uneducated and unskilled women often drawn from among the inmates of the latter.

In the newly established teaching hospitals women were trained under hierarchical organisations of matron, sister, nurses, helpers, watchers. On-the-spot training was provided for higher ranks and promotions were usually made from the ranks. In Catholic countries nursing orders were augmented by volunteer parish women, who were expected to call in a nurse if they considered it necessary.

When the well-to-do fled the towns during the plague of 1665–6, their physicians often fleeing with them, servants frequently remained, hiring out their services as nurses in order to gain a living. These nurses frequently cared for the sick with outstanding courage, skill and devotion: but some resorted to robbery and violence amongst their helpless charges, gaining for nurses at large an evil reputation.

The position of hospital nurses during the eighteenth and first half of the nineteenth century remained degraded for two main reasons: on the one hand, untrained and destitute persons were increasingly brought in to save expenses; on the other, male medical students were increasingly allowed on womens' wards, taking from nurses their more skilled and medically interesting work, thus making it necessary to readjust the boundaries between nursing and medicine.

Growing feeling that the sick had a right to medical treatment and doctors a right to payment for services provided to all patient groups was a blow to ideas of nursing as a calling of dedication to be rewarded by compliance and gratitude. Apart from those working in hospitals through their attachment to religious orders, educated women did not usually nurse the hospitalised sick. Those dedicated to the care of the latter for spiritual reasons were accustomed to unquestioning acceptance of discipline imposed from above, whatever its nature. Nurses from lower classes of society lacked the skill and training to be placed in positions of responsibility and pay was too low to make nursing a profitable career. When religious orders were abolished it was stipulated by the Government of the day that individuals already looking after the poor should continue to do so under the supervision of local government administrators; but *new* nurses of high calibre were not available. At the end of the eighteenth century nurses were still being recruited without training and prior investigation as to suitability for the work involved. Consequently, standards were often appalling.

In Poor Law institutions nurses were usually required to live in and to attend their patients by night as well as by day. In addition to attending to personal needs they were expected to perform tasks (such as the scrubbing of floors) traditionally those of low-grade servants. Drunkenness was common amongst them (a daily ration of a pint or more of porter, and one or two glasses of gin for night duty and especially disagreeable work was permitted). Local attempts at reform met with little success for reasons of lack of interest from a public in whose view hospitals were only for paupers, soldiers and sufferers from epidemic diseases.

Florence Nightingale

'. . . There is a growing conviction that in all hospitals, even in those which are best conducted, there is a great and unnecessary waste of life: and that, as a general rule, the poor would recover better in their own miserable dwellings if they had proper medical and surgical aid, and efficient nursing, than they do under more refined treatment in hospitals. But few have so sad or so large an experience as I have had to lead them to this conviction' (Florence Nightingale, *Notes on Hospitals*, 1863 (rev.)).

Miss Nightingale had learned from personal experience that, in addition to tenderness and patience, good nursing requires ample knowledge, skill, discipline and organisation. In these views she found herself in conflict on two sides: on one, with the medical profession, which wanted to exclude nurses from all but roles subordinate to medicine; on the other, with nurses who objected to working within an established framework, under instruction and supervision, but who, nevertheless, were frequently more knowledgeable about the needs of their patients than were doctors themselves.

Perhaps the most significant of Miss Nightingale's achieve-

ments for the nursing profession as a whole was autonomy in
matters of formation and training. However, recognising dangers
for patients inherent in circumstances where nurses frequently
changed or supplemented treatments prescribed by doctors, she
gained formal acceptance of requirements that nurses *must* work
according to medical prescriptions. This pleased the medical
profession but upset many nurses who sought professional
autonomy in all respects.[10]

District nursing

Professional home nursing as an alternative to hospital admission
has never been available in Britain other than to the wealthy.
Organisational reform in its favour has always lagged behind
that in favour of hospitals because the mainstream of medicine
has always been hospital orientated.

In 1840 a social reformer, Elizabeth Fry, established an
Institute of Nursing in London for the training of women in home
nursing. These women first called themselves Protestant Sisters of
Charity. But, in response to feeling against church interference in
secular affairs, a change in name to that of 'Nursing Sisters' was
made. Applicants were carefully selected for personal qualities
and nursing aptitude, then trained – initially at Guy's Hospital in
London. The Institute paid their salaries and acted as a registry;
money for their pay came from donations and contributions from
patients. These Sisters wore uniforms and their work was closely
supervised by the Institute.[11]

In 1859 a district nursing service was founded in Liverpool,
through the establishment of a Training School and Home for
Nurses, in co-operation with Liverpool Royal Infirmary. This led
to an investigation into conditions in workhouses, now filled with
sick persons receiving little or no proper nursing care. The ill
effects of Poor Law legislation, which obliged the sick to accept
indoor rather than outdoor relief, had become increasingly
apparent to public authorities, who, nevertheless, were financially inhibited from making alternative domiciliary arrangements. It was not until the ending of the Poor Law and the
creation of the NHS that home nursing became an integral part
of statutory health provision. Even since then, however, it has

remained very much a piecemeal service, relying largely on vague notions of co-ordination and liaison with other (statutory and voluntary) bodies interested in the home care of the sick and handicapped, for items not of a specifically skilled nursing nature.

Midwives

At first sight it might be thought that a profession concerned with the natural process of childbirth would be irrelevant in a book concerned with the care of the sick. Closer examination, however, makes clear that this is not the case. The history of midwifery is crucial to the consideration of domiciliary provision for the sick for three reasons: first, the medical profession includes midwifery in obstetrics, one of three essential branches of general medicine; second, there is a place for a domiciliary midwifery service based on concepts similar to, but not identical with, those applying to 'hospital at home' for sick persons; third, where illness accompanies childbirth, services similar to the latter, but also capable of incorporating midwifery, might offer mother and child better prospects of recovery and safe delivery than would admission to hospital.

Legislation in 1858 deprived midwives of rights of practice independent from the medical profession by decreeing midwifery to be an integral part of medicine. Doctors saw midwives as nurses, specialised in childbirth, who would be at hand to perform tasks which they themselves did not wish to perform. However, they had no objection to their continued operation amongst the lower classes whose members could not afford medical fees.[12]

In many ways sick nurses gained from their subordination to doctors, which at least offered them prospects of secure, if not lucrative, livings. Educated midwives, on the other hand, already enjoyed relatively secure, financially rewarding and professionally satisfying lives. But when doctors gained experience in the lying-in rooms of hospitals it became fashionable for women of the upper classes to hire them in preference to women midwives qualified to practice alone. The latter, who had hitherto enjoyed the patronage of a clientele able to pay them well for their services, objected to having to relinquish this to the medical profession. But others not so fortunate were happy to accept the subordinate role of midwifery nurses, which offered them benefits similar to those of nurses of the sick. Competent midwives of all persuasions were, however, cognisant of the need to call upon medical help when it seemed that a birth was not proceeding normally.[13]

A series of measures and counter-measures between doctors and midwives and respective groups of the latter left midwives outside hospitals largely to their own devices until the beginning of the twentieth century. But, as doctors gained from growing public interest in medical intervention in childbirth, educated midwives, who objected in principle to being used as midwifery nurses, found themselves under increasing threat of extinction. They were, however, in an extraordinarily difficult position, for reasons of the large number of uneducated colleagues in their midsts, some of whom, although often highly knowledgeable about childbirth (having experienced it themselves or amongst women of their neighbourhoods on many occasions), were often given to unwarranted and dangerous interference in birth processes.[14] They would have liked to see the introduction of compulsory registration, subject to satisfaction of minimum requirements; but this would have resulted in depriving a large section of the population of midwifery assistance of any kind, particularly in areas where there were no lying-in hospitals. Thus they were torn between desire for professional development and the need to ensure availability of assistance to all women of all classes and circumstances.[15]

In 1882 the Matrons' Aid Society was set up, to be re-designated a few years later the Midwives' Institute. In 1902 a Midwives Act was passed, representing a severe and public humiliation for the General Medical Council, British Medical Association and other medical bodies, at the hands of womens' organisations, Parliament and the Government. This Act confirmed full professional status for qualified midwives who, by law, were not now to be called midwifery or obstetric nurses; laying foundations for present-day midwives' regulations (as formulated in the Act of 1951). However, it had the effect of placing midwives at a disadvantage amongst both doctors and nurses: first, in conferring upon them state registration, it subjected them to local authority supervision usually associated with the licensing of tradespeople; second, professional misconduct leading to liability to erasure from the Register was widely and minutely defined and included the right of their disciplinary body to enquire into their private lives; third, in contrast with other professions, midwifery was not to be allowed self-regulation – indeed a rival (the medical profession) was to have the dominant voice in its government.[16]

The end of an era

Throughout the nineteenth century hospitals, the Poor Law, doctors, nurses and midwives operated largely without regard for the health needs of the population as a whole. Their concern was for individuals presently under their care, the protection of their institutions, professional gain and/or personal advancement. Such an approach was totally unsuited to public needs in circumstances where the industrial population had increased from around 7 million at the beginning of the century to over 40 million in the 1870s. The growth of clubs and friendly societies providing sickness insurance for workers and health and sanitary reform, spurred on by the outbreak of two cholera epidemics and the birth of the trade union movement in the latter half of the century, aroused public feeling in favour of more universal and egalitarian health provision. By the end of the century Britain was ready for radical reforms which would ultimately lead to the creation of a national health service. This, when it came, was to set seal against the involvement of GPs in hospital medicine and that of hospital specialists in the treatment of patients at home.

References

(1) Woodward, J., *To Do the Sick no Harm*, Routledge and Keegan Paul, London, 1974, pp. 2–3.

(2) Pollak, K., *The Healers*, Nelson, London, 1968, pp. 94–9.

(3) Woodward, *op. cit.*, p. 27.

(4) Abel-Smith, B., *The Hospitals 1800–1948*, Heinemann, London, 1964, pp. 101–18.

(5) *Ibid.*, p. 95.

(6) *Ibid.*, pp. 119–32.

(7) Honigsbaum, F., *The Division in British Medicine*, Kogan Page, London, 1979, pp. 13–14.

(8) Bullough, V. L., and Bullough, B., *The Care of the Sick*, Croom Helm, London, 1979, pp. 38–43.

(9) Abel-Smith, B., *History of the Nursing Profession*, Heinemann, London, 1960, pp. 1–16.

(10) Abel-Smith, *The Hospitals 1800–1948*, *op. cit.*, pp. 66–82.

(11) Bullough and Bullough, *op. cit.* pp. 80–1.

(12) Donnison, J., *Midwives and Medical Men*, Schocken Books, New York, 1977, pp. 88–115.

(13) *Ibid.*

(14) Shorter, E., *A History of Women's Bodies*, Basic Books, New York, 1982, and Allen Lane, London, 1983.

(15) Donnison, *op. cit.*, p. 177.

(16) *Ibid.*, pp. 174–5.

2 Foundations of modern health care in Britain: a divided medical service and consequences for the sick

Introduction

Attempts at the introduction of a national health policy in Britain had been made in the nineteenth century. In 1848 a General Board of Health was set up, followed by a Local Government Board in 1871. Both collapsed in the face of medical opposition, although the latter continued to hold minimal powers until stripped of functions and bypassed by the creation of other departments.[1]

New attitudes towards the care of the sick were partly due to reforms of the Local Government Act of 1894, which altered the constitution of Poor Law Boards of Guardians – sweeping away financial qualifications, abolishing *ex-officio* Guardians, and enabling the appointment of married women who were encouraged to become members of visiting committees. These reforms led to new attitudes to the poor and the realisation that the preaching of thrift to 'people who had nothing to be thrifty about'[2] was futile. By the turn of the century it was clear that the Poor Law in its existing form was an anachronism and would have to be replaced by legislation more suited to modern-day needs and aspirations.

National insurance

Evidence from the Royal Commission on Poor Laws (1905–9) pointed to unco-ordinated, haphazard development of hospital facilities as an area of major health concern. Reform in this respect was certain to be hampered, since neither voluntary nor local authority hospital bodies were likely to be willing to relinquish respective holds unless circumstances from outside forced them to do so. Meanwhile, better means of care than were presently possible for the sick poor in their own homes were urgently required. The solution favoured by a majority report of the Commission was to make facilities of sickness insurance available to as many people as possible and to provide a residual service for those unable to pay the necessary premiums.[3]

GPs largely welcomed the National Health Insurance (NHI) Act of 1911, because it enabled them to escape the unpleasant necessity to meet conditions laid down by the representatives of tradespeople and/or their employees in their former panel work. Despite the fact that the Act made no provision for the families of workers, and indeed failed to provide for a large section of the working population itself, it furthered the idea of family doctoring but strengthened GP opposition against health centre development, a concept widely supported in progressive circles.[4]

Until the passing of the NHI Act, public pressure, backed by a number of public-spirited doctors, for the appointment of a Ministry of Health which would co-ordinate all health care activities had been steadily gaining ground. The introduction of national health insurance weakened this pressure because the medical profession gained from the NHI Act many advantages it thought it would accrue from a Ministry of Health. However, as the limitations of insurance became increasingly apparent, pressure for more universal provision once more gained in strength. At the time public feeling had been aroused by the appallingly high rate of infant mortality in the country, which, of all public health indices, had failed to fall in the nineteenth century and indeed had begun to rise at the beginning of the twentieth.[5]

The main body of the medical profession was not opposed to

state intervention in all health matters. In general, doctors welcomed it as a means of action in their favour when they did not wish to, or could not, take action themselves. With voluntary hospitals outside the orbit of statutory control and problems resulting from lack of co-ordination between public and voluntary hospitals (or between one voluntary hospital and another) there were many aspects of patient or professional interest in which they were unable to take effective action.

The 1914–18 war

The tendency of Poor Law and municipal services towards the employment of salaried doctors effectively blocked private practitioner involvement in local authority work. Hospital specialists were not affected by the provisions of the NHI Act. Their private practices were assured through their voluntary and teaching hospital appointments which brought private custom in their wake. With the outbreak of the 1914–18 war GPs assumed that their presence would from then on be required in local authority hospitals (enabling their access to hospital resources and clinical facilities, essential to good standards of practice in both their panel and their private work). They were to be disappointed. Although their presence in hospitals proved indispensable when *all* available medical services were required for the treatment of the war-wounded, GPs became redundant when casualties dropped in number and newly qualified doctors were recruited to hospital posts in large numbers direct from their medical schools. This left specialists free to select doctors who would work under rather than in co-operation with them. Meanwhile, GPs were faced with panel practices depleted by military call-up; threats of a spread of state medicine through the appointment of salaried local authority doctors for the non-insured; and the growth of hospital out-patient departments, which further depleted demand for their private services.

The desperate search for beds for war-wounded service personnel had a dramatic effect on hospital development. At first, both military and civilian patients were obliged to accept

hospital accommodation wherever it could be found. Doctors
and nurses found themselves working in types of hospitals quite
different from those they would have contemplated had there
been no war. Within each hospital there might be wide
discrepancies in the pay of both doctors and nurses because
allocation had taken place via different employing authorities.
When in 1916 there was a lull in fighting and the number of
casualties fell dramatically, thousands of beds in voluntary
hospitals reserved for Services patients fell vacant, while civilians
could not get treatment. Instead of being redeployed for the use
of the latter, these beds were then redistributed to Services
personnel according to rank, nationality and colour – officers
receiving the most choice accommodation – an affront to egalitarian concepts emerging from the events of war. This brought
home to Parliament a crucial need for health reform directed
towards the lasting protection of the civilian population, reviving
pressure for a Ministry of Health (MOH) under central and local
democratic control.[6]

Ministry of Health

It was originally anticipated that MOH services would be run
from hospitals to which, where possible, public health services
would be transferred. The notion was that hospitals would
provide 'health centres', including in-patient accommodation,
whereby preventive and curative sectors of medicine would be
brought together. Had hospital specialists desired the presence of
GPs in hospitals it is likely that the health centre idea might have
become the foundation for future health provision: but by now
teaching hospital practice of patient care through medical 'firms'
headed by consultants had gained the support of the most
powerful sections of the organised medical profession. It was
essential, therefore, to the interests of the profession as a whole,
that GPs should be found a role independent of hospital work.
This specialists conceived for them in the field of prevention.[7]

Having lost their battle for access to hospitals, GPs were
obliged to consider their futures in terms of community work

alone. Any interest they might have felt in medical cover for the population through taxation rather than insurance was countered by fears of interference in their private practices from local medical officers of health. Contract work with state-approved insurance bodies at least protected them from this. Meanwhile, deprived of access to around half their supply of doctors and a third of the hospital beds,[8] and with state insurance covering only part of the working population and none of its families, public demand for comprehensive medical cover grew. By the beginning of the 1920s the idea had been accepted in principle, but agreement had not been reached by the medical profession as to the form it should take in practice.

Three distinct bodies of doctors were by now involved in public health administration: first, in the operation of the Poor Law; second, in the municipal health system; third, in the operation of the panel system. Theoretically, private practitioners could serve all three bodies. But, since none now offered the prospect of hospital work, GPs effectively had a straight choice between non-hospital practice under salaried service, headed by local medical officers of health, or non-hospital practice under independent contract to approved insurance societies, with the prospect of expanding private practice where insurance cover was not available for patients. The majority chose the latter. Thus prospects of a national health service, very much alive in the minds of progressive professional and lay circles after the 1914–18 war, were delayed for over a quarter of a century, due largely to wrangling between divisions within the medical profession rather than to rooted objections from outside.

In 1919 the British Labour Party published a report favouring the setting up of a Ministry of Health, which would provide personal health and social services through health centres. The report assumed that these health centres would be based on public hospitals throughout the country. A later report by the Trades Union Congress and Labour Party published in 1922 enlarges on the concept thus:

' . . . a completely organised hospital service, with receiving stations, cottage hospitals, county hospitals, and national hospitals, ramifying throughout the length and breadth of the country, all working together for the speedy cure of individual sufferers and for raising the standard of health of the whole nation. Each hospital should become the "Health Centre" of the district which it serves. . . . '[9]

(This concept is of crucial significance to *Hospital at Home*.)

A Ministry of Health was set up in the spring of 1919, taking over functions from the Board of Control, Insurance Commissioners, Privy Council, Board of Education and Local Government Board. The Act setting up the ministry empowered the establishment of consultative committees, a power which was used to establish a Council on Medical and Administrative Services, chaired by Sir Bertrand Dawson, a prominent physician of the day. This Council was asked by the Minister of Health to consider 'the scheme or schemes requisite for the systematised provisions of such forms of medical and allied services as should, in the opinion of the Council, be available for the inhabitants of a given area'.[10]

The Dawson Report of 1920[11] was a revolutionary document, bearing remarkable similarities to the Labour Party report published two years earlier. It largely ignored previous historical developments, underlying philosophies and the existing framework to medical care in Britain: instead it started from first principles and then, where possible, suggested the incorporation of existing medical services into its plans.

There were, however, important differences between Labour Party plans and those put forward by the Dawson Report. While the former envisaged that doctors would be entirely based on health centres, the latter envisaged that GPs would continue to run their surgeries from their own homes, with their accommodation in health centres to be tried only where local medical opinion favoured it. Furthermore, it was opposed to a full-time salaried service.

The Dawson Report foresaw a division in Britain's health services between those of a primary and those of a secondary nature. This division was not to give rise to separate hospital and community sectors. Primary health centres were to provide simple health services and were to be staffed by GPs aided by visiting consultants: they would include hospital beds. More difficult patient-cases or those requiring more specialised treatment were to be passed on to secondary health centres, staffed mainly by consultants and specialists, but not excluding GPs.

While the model of health care described in the Dawson Report was under discussion, problems more pressing for the medical profession arose in the voluntary hospital sector, which appeared to be on the verge of collapse. In the face of severe financial difficulties, many voluntary hospitals had abandoned their traditions of free treatment, and all over the country various schemes for making charges were introduced. The Ministry of Health was drawn into the search for solutions, one of its suggestions being that local authorities should be allowed to subscribe to voluntary hospitals – a suggestion rejected by the medical profession on the grounds that it would curtail its own powers over hospitals not already under local authority control.[12]

Debate on the future of voluntary hospitals had the effect of weakening support for proposals of the Dawson Report favouring nationalisation; and these were dropped when the Ministry of Health (Miscellaneous Provisions) Bill was presented to the House of Commons in 1920.[13] This meant that the Poor Law, thought to have been doomed at the end of the 1914–18 war, would have to be retained. Although Boards of Guardians were abolished in 1929, it was not until the creation of the National Health Service (NHS) in 1948 that non-means-tested universal medical cover was finally to be made available in Britain.

The 1939–44 war

Gaining from lessons learned during the 1914–18 war, the Ministry of Health had prepared well ahead for a war which was generally accepted as inevitable by the late 1930s. At its outbreak in 1939, it might have been expected that the services of GPs would again, as before, be required in hospitals to deal with casualties (this time including the victims of air-raids), especially as the Ministry of Health had only around 3500 fully qualified specialists stationed in hospitals under its control. This, however, the Department refused to allow – the division between hospital and community services, reinforced by the attitude of the British Medical Association (BMA), now being organisationally complete. Instead, it resolved problems of doctor shortage by spreading more evenly across the country the available supply of consultant services and giving them powers to act on their own.[14]

In 1939 an Emergency Medical Service was set up, recruiting from all hospital medical grades (house officer to consultant), and thus avoiding the need to call upon GPs from outside. In reality the Emergency Medical Service was uniquely a hospital service which further reinforced exclusion by specialists of GP access to hospital beds.[15]

When proposals for a national health service were once more put before the country immediately following the war, the range of treatment and quality of care in general practice remained as low as it had been in the 1930s.[16] Meanwhile modern scientific and technological advances, whose widespread application in hospitals had been spurred on by the consequences of war, made massive expenditure on its hospital sector at the expense of its community services inevitable. GPs were therefore glad to be assured of financial security through *per capita* payments covering the whole population, instead of, as previously, insured workers alone; independent contracts offering them freedom to interpret their roles largely according to standards set by themselves; and opportunities for private practice outside their NHS work. When the NHS finally came into operation in 1948, they had already abandoned ambitions they might previously have had in the direction of hospital practice.

An inside view of hospitals prior to the creation of the NHS

Since the impressions of hospitals held by many people, the elderly in particular, are in part related to experiences of pre-NHS days, this chapter would not be complete without an attempt to convey some of these impressions to readers lacking experience of their own upon which to draw. Many hospital units of today are sited in old buildings, lacking modern amenities, often reflecting outdated concepts and attitudes towards patients care. It helps in the understanding of fears which frequently accompany hospital admission to know something of the memories that these old buildings may hold.

My own impressions of hospitals date back to childhood. I was five years old when my two year old brother was admitted to the district hospital some 20 miles away from home. Visiting was not allowed, so my father had crept alongside the ward where he lay in the hope of gaining a glimpse of him. He described how he had found him, strapped flat on his back following an operation, alone and unaided, trying to eat jelly off a tea-plate. It seemed insufferable that a place where people went to be made better could overlook so important a problem of daily living!

Or, I remember how an aunt suffering pernicious anaemia spent her last months in a crowded sick ward of the local workhouse because no other hospital would accept her case; how my mother, with five young children, struggled to care for her senile incontinent father, rather than have him admitted to the same place. I also recall that use of the local cottage hospital was monopolised (so my mother said) by 'the other GP' in the town – he being the one with a flourishing private practice – while our own family doctor was obliged to resort to the Poor Law infirmary for his patients if their home care proved impossible.

Personally, I had little to do with hospitals until 1939, when I came to London to work as a medical superintendent's clerk. From this position it was possible to gain insight into wide and varied aspects of hospital life, from both patient and staff viewpoints.

Each London County Council (LCC) hospital was headed by a medical superintendent. He was responsible for all clinical services in the hospital. The matron looked after domestic and nursing affairs, the steward oversaw general administration. There were about 500 beds in our hospital, over which the medical superintendent, assisted by a resident physician and surgeon and perhaps six or seven house doctors, held unique control. Visiting specialists from London's teaching hospitals attended on sessional bases, sometimes bringing with them their students.

In our hospital (an ex-Poor Law infirmary) there were two
medical superintendent's clerks who between them filled the
roles of receptionist, admissions clerk, records and transport
officer, and medical secretary. Our work brought us into contact
with virtually all sections of hospital personnel and a wide variety
of health and welfare personnel from outside – GPs, Poor Law
relieving officers, visiting specialists, local chest clinic and
dispensary nurses, ambulance drivers, to name but a few – and a
constant stream of visits from patient's relatives, usually in
connection with cases of serious illness or death.

Thus we came to know a great deal about public attitudes to
local authority hospitals viz à viz those towards voluntary and
teaching hospitals. In our easy accessibility to all who set foot
inside the hospital (our office was in the main entrance hall near
the casualty department) we learned much of the anxieties of
hospital experiences which beset health professionals and those
whom they serve.

Patients of the early 1940s still had good reason to fear hospital
admission, if only for the dangers it held of loss of employment or
home: neither of which were then usually protected as they are
today. The possibility that application for Poor Law relief
necessitated by a hospital admission might lead to a dreaded
move to the workhouse (or 'institution' as it was now officially
known) discouraged sick wage-earners from seeking medical
help and their families from seeking social and financial help to
tide them over difficult times.

The 60-bed wards in our hospital were subdivided into five
bays – the fifth of which held long-stay patients not fit enough to
be sent home or transferred to the nearby institution. At the time
it was LCC policy to up-grade the better institutions under its
administration, with the aim of transferring to them as many as
possible of the chronically sick patients who blocked the beds of
municipal hospitals aspiring to 'general acute' designation.
Patients of the fifth bay dreaded a visit from the relieving officer
to determine whether they might be transferred to the nearby
workhouse, sometimes feigning acute illness in the hope that they
would be judged unfit to be moved. Outside private and
voluntary sectors, there were no elderly persons' homes. Neither
were domiciliary services, such as those of home helps and meals
on wheels, available at the time. District nursing services were

abysmally inadequate and in any case not yet under direct statutory control.

Although, as a designated general hospital, ours admitted a complement of acutely ill patients, the nearby presence of voluntary and teaching hospitals ensured that our cases would usually be those of a type rejected by the latter. Furthermore, doctors of the latter were able to transfer to us patients no longer of medical interest to themselves. Consequently our reputation as a hospital offering good prospects of recovery suffered, making it yet more difficult to escape an image largely created throughout years of operation as a Poor Law institution.

Many marked differences between voluntary and teaching hospitals and those of the kind in which I worked during the early 1940s were related to nursing provision. Teaching hospitals were able to recruit from long waiting lists of would-be nurses, mainly drawn from well educated, socially advantaged groups of society. LCC hospitals were obliged to recruit mainly from areas where there was a plentiful supply of young girls seeking to leave home, perhaps to gain employment or escape poor and over-crowded conditions. As I recall, around 40 per cent of nurses in our hospital were from Ireland. Although, ill-paid, nursing offered security, accommodation, and prospects of gaining qualification in a now highly respected profession. Nurses who did not leave (usually to get married) during their probation years were frequently promoted to senior posts, passing on to new recruits experience gained and practices adopted during their own in-training. Following qualification, teaching-hospital nurses tended to remain where they had trained or else to move on to voluntary hospitals. But they seldom opted for work in local authority institutions. There is nothing to suggest that our nurses were any the less disciplined, caring and dedicated in their work than were nurses in teaching hospitals: but their backgrounds, together with staff shortages which did not apply in the latter, and the type of patient-case with which they traditionally had to cope, ensured that the position of local authority hospital nurses would remain degraded until status differences between teaching and voluntary hospitals on the one hand, state hospitals on the other, should disappear.

It must be difficult for anyone who has not in person experienced work in hospitals from pre-NHS days onwards to appreciate changes which have taken place and obstacles in the way of change encountered in them. Theoretically such changes could have taken place with the introduction of modern treatments and techniques which immediately followed the war years. In practice, some outdated ideas and customs have persisted, and even today lie behind common causes of patient unhappiness. Patient visiting, for example, although now much less restricted than it was in early NHS days, is still regarded by many nurses as an unwarranted interruption of ward routines.

In the 1940s visitors would queue in the street outside our hospital twice a week, awaiting the bell which heralded the opening of the main gates. As I remember, visiting time lasted only an hour. No children were allowed to visit and the rule for adults was varied only in 'danger-list' cases. I well remember the nursing outcry when a progressively-minded paediatrician tried to introduce visiting in the children's wards just prior to the introduction of the NHS! Staff were convinced this would cause upset endangering the lives of their young charges and make their proper nursing care impossible.

In retrospect, it is often difficult to determine which hospital restrictions in common practice in the early days of the NHS were necessary in the interests of patients themselves and which were outdated legacies from the past. Health authorities under central government now assumed responsibility for hospital as well as community services in their areas. They were committed to policies of control over the spread of infection among the public as a whole as well as that among their warded patients. And, as all NHS hospitals would henceforth be used by patients of all classes, strict discipline had to be observed to raise and maintain high standards.

Widespread programmes of public innoculation against infectious diseases were not usually well under way until the mid-1950s. Tuberculosis was still rife and often devastating in its effects. The use of antibiotics was still restricted and limited in potential. Warded patients had to be protected from cross-infections and the introduction of epidemic diseases from outside.

Thus, rigid policies of staff and patient control which would not be tolerated today might then have been essential. For example, patients in general wards were not usually allowed out of bed, even when quite capable of walking around. This necessitated seemingly unending ward rounds of one kind or another: bedpan; washing; bedmaking; meals. At the same time, it is difficult to understand, for example, why it still should have been so important to ensure that the wheels of all the beds should be set at the same angle in readiness for a visit from the matron or some other dignitary!

It must also be recalled that in the 1940s and early 1950s many labour-saving devices taken for granted in hospitals today were then unheard of, unobtainable or in short supply. At the same time, there was no shortage of cheap, unskilled, female labour, unprotected by union legislation. Consequently many hospital practices and routines were determined by the presence of armies of cleaners and domestics who had to satisfy the eagle eye of the matron as to the pristine state of her domain. This must surely have interfered with the freedom of patients to move freely as they do today around hospital wards, corridors and grounds.

Most of us of the third and fourth generations who worked in or were patients of hospitals in early NHS days will have experienced conditions similar to those described above. As a result we may hold reservations about hospital life which are not by and large shared with members of later generations. But we are sharply reminded how outdated and now unacceptable practices persist or are revived, when evidence of them sometimes comes to light following public complaint.

Whatever individual feelings about hospitals may be, lessons of the past are surely that patients should not be admitted to them unless this is crucial for treatment reasons. It therefore seems logical that health policies should be directed at extending as far as possible arrangements for the home care of the sick. This cannot happen unless and until medical, nursing and social skills, general and specialist, are integrated outside as well as inside hospitals. It has long been recognised, even in hospitals, that families of the sick have an important part to play in the recovery and general well-being of the latter. Where home care is involved, however, it is crucial that health authorities should develop policies capable of incorporating fully the willing and able contributions of families, friends and neighbours, according to sensitive assessment of the needs and possibilities of each individual case.

References

(1) Honigsbaum, F., *The Division of British Medicine*, Kogan Page, London, 1979, p. 22.
(2) Abel-Smith, B., *The Hospitals, 1800–1948*, Heinemann, London, 1964, p. 201.
(3) *Ibid.*, pp. 217–32.
(4) Honigsbaum, *op. cit.*, pp. 9–21.
(5) *Ibid.*, pp. 22–41.
(6) Abel-Smith, *op. cit.*, pp. 267–283.
(7) Honigsbaum, *op. cit.*, pp. 137–149.
(8) Abel-Smith, *op. cit.*, pp. 282–3.
(9) *Ibid.*, p. 319.
(10) *Ibid.*, p. 289.
(11) Honigsbaum, *op. cit.*, pp. 64–72.
(12) Abel-Smith, *op. cit.*, pp. 284–302.
(13) *Ibid.*, p. 299.
(14) Honigsbaum, *op. cit.*, p. 173.
(15) *Ibid.*, p. 173.
(16) *Ibid.*, pp. 150–61, 233.

3 The National Health Service: high dependency patients at home – the case for a secondary domiciliary care service

The Beveridge Report on social insurance (1942) proposed the extension and co-ordination of existing social insurance schemes on the assumption that a comprehensive national health service would be required to achieve medical objectives envisaged in the Report. Beveridge took the view that social insurance should cover all income groups and their dependents. But he regarded restoration of a sick person to health as a duty of the state prior to any other consideration. Events of the 1939–44 war (like that of 1914–18) had concerted public opinion in favour of widespread changes which would promote greater social justice and equality in Britain. Consequently, the Beveridge Report was greeted with enthusiasm such as had never before and has never since been experienced when proposals for social reform have been made.[1]

The years between publication of the Report and the passing of the National Health Service Act (1946) were fraught with controversy, chiefly concerning the conditions under which the medical profession would participate in the Service. The question of GP involvement in hospital work, however, hardly arose. Only GPs with access to nursing and convalescent homes by now received payment for bed-cases, presumably because they were virtually the only units where specialists had no particular claim to beds. Few such units had facilities suitable for the treatment of the acutely ill and even if they had it would only have been a matter of time before scientific and technological advances would make them obsolete. Already a source of pay-beds, which for a significant group of GPs had provided a vested interest in the hospital sector, was in danger of drying up. Patients were turning from nursing homes and pay-beds in cottage hospitals to pay-beds under specialist control in the voluntary hospitals, which in turn stimulated public interest in provident schemes from which GPs were largely excluded.[2]

Despite a vigorous campaign from within the ranks of the BMA (led by Dr E. R. Fothergill, who himself owned a nursing home) supporting NHS provision of nursing home access for GPs, the possibility was ignored by the BMA, whose independent Medical Planning Commission set up in 1940 produced a working document in anticipation of the Beveridge Report and NHS proposals.[3] When Dawson (of the 1920 Dawson Report) opened the proceedings of the first meeting of the Commission he stressed the need for all doctors, including GPs, to participate in hospital work. However, apparently, after this first meeting he took no further part in the Commission's activities, passing the lead to a public health representative (Dr Buchan, Medical Officer of Health for Willesden) who immediately orientated it in favour of community care, predicting that it would find the role of GPs in the NHS the most difficult of its problems to resolve.

Taken together, the Beveridge Report and the BMA Commission's Report conceived for the NHS its final form on its creation in 1948. This did provide the nation with universal medical cover, free of charge at the time of need, as was the aim of its architect, Aneurin Bevan. But, in conceding universal cover to GPs under independent contract to health authorities, instead of through salaried services, and in conceding to the BMA view that GPs should not have access to hospital facilities, Bevan failed in his ambition to integrate hospital and community facilities within an organisation capable of response according to the particular needs of each patient's case. Whether or not Government concessions to a divided medical profession were a necessary condition for the creation of the NHS in 1948 can probably never be known. Certainly they were fundamental to many of the seemingly intractable problems experienced in its organisation ever since that time. Nevertheless, the creation of the NHS was a milestone as a measure of co-ordination and rationalisation, following many years of largely unplanned development in the health field. It also signified a new era of state acceptance of responsibility for comprehensive health and welfare – even if it did not provide successive Governments with powers to meet that responsibility in full.

A widely held belief that shortcomings of the NHS could be overcome by improvements in levels and varieties of resources alone has not been borne out in practice over the past three decades. Where health is concerned it is unlikely that supply could ever meet demand, so resource allocations must be made according to priorities. These are difficult to determine in circumstances where they vary according to different interests amongst both professional and lay groups. So health authorities usually direct them to hospital sectors, where the demand and case made for their use is most powerful and where they can best control and monitor their use. Where a community sector does attract additional resources these tend to be swallowed into an amorphous mass of services incapable of assuring their effective use. Even where individuals responsible for their allocation are themselves satisfied in this respect, they lack means of demonstrating it to their employers.

Under its existing organisation the NHS never has been and never will be capable of ensuring optimum use of resources outside its hospital sector. This presents a serious dilemma for patients requiring specialist treatment and high levels and wide varieties of support services, but not, essentially, hospital beds: also for health authorities for whom the last mentioned are in short supply.

From the creation of the NHS onward certain concepts fundamental to its effective planning appear to have been ignored by those responsible. They concern terms in everyday use, or mis-use, according to which provisions are traditionally made and their consumers identified. Foremost of these terms is that of 'a patient'.[4] Until GP panel practices were introduced the term applied only to a person undergoing treatment from a doctor. But when GPs built up their practices, first through sickness insurance arrangements, later through universal medical cover provided by the NHS, a custom arose whereby even fit persons were known as 'panel' or 'list' patients of some GP or another. This inspired notions that treatment services outside hospitals should be organised around groups including both fit and sick persons. This fitted well with the preventive roles conceived by specialists for GPs and accepted by the latter when

they finally abandoned hope of involvement in the hospital
sector. However, it created confusion about the often disparate
needs of the healthy to remain fit and the sick to be made better.

Undoubtedly, persons admitted to hospitals are patients. As
such their treatment, care and basic support are the responsibility of these hospitals. Outside, where virtually everyone is the list
patient of some GP or another, there is no clear-cut distinction
between persons undergoing treatment and the rest of the
population. It is therefore impossible to organise services which
take into proper account care and support needs necessary to
enable optimum effective treatment. Inevitably, health authorities must be bound by the clinical requirements of individual
GPs. This being the case, it is out of the question that they should
develop their community health sectors in favour of high levels
and wide varieties of patient care, unless and until persons
potentially entitled to them can be clearly identified. This can
occur only if GP services become the responsibility of health
authorities and preventive services are separated from those of
treatment.

Because, it is assumed, GPs provide preventive, early diagnostic and minor treatment services, but not those required in
cases of major illness, they have come to be regarded as heads of
'primary health care teams'. The extent of such teamwork as
actually takes place depends largely on individual GP initiative.
Much of it, however, is inevitably concentrated on cases which
are not of a primary kind. These concern patients suffering
major – secondary or terminal – illness. When the care of such
patients becomes too much for their families, perhaps with
limited help from primary care services, they have to be
hospitalised. Thus, an artificial distinction is made, which, *de
facto*, equates major illness with need for institutionalisation. For
many the consequences of separation from home and family and
loss of human dignity are disastrous.

The NHS was originally based on a tripartite system made up
as follows: hospital divisions staffed by salaried doctors; GPs
under independent contracts; community health and welfare
under local government (MOH) administration. Major reorganisation, effected in 1974, avoided any move which would
have brought GP services within the orbit of health authority
administration.

In 1971, following recommendations of the Seebohm Report,[5] local government services were reorganised to provide an umbrella service designed to cover all aspects of social need.[6] Seebohm left open to speculation how the work of the NHS might be affected by his recommendations.

The idea behind the ending of the tripartite system was described by Richard Crossman, first Secretary of State in the new Department of Health and Social Services (DHSS) set up following the Social Service Act (1970).

'Unification', said Crossman, 'offers solid advantages to the individual and the family, because their needs for health and social services are not divided into separate compartments. A single family, or an individual, may in a short time, or even at one and the same time, need many types of health and social care, and these needs should be met in a co-ordinated way. Otherwise they will get an unsatisfactory service or even no service at all.'[7]

With such high ideals behind them it might have been expected that the reorganisations which took place in the early 1970s would have realised dramatic and immediate improvements in health and welfare provision. This was not the case. In the first place NHS reorganisation was delayed by four years due to failure on the part of successive Governments of the time to produce plans acceptable to all interested parties, in particular the medical profession. When the Act was finally passed in 1973 it confirmed that GPs would retain their independent status and that specialists would retain an exclusive hold on hospital medicine. The appointment of physicians as heads of community divisions of health authority districts did not achieve a hoped for integration of community patient services because the latter, being mainly GP services, were outside their orbits of control. As hospital sectors remained separate from those of the community, far from being ended by reorganisation, the tripartite system was thereby reinforced.

In the General Election of 1970 Labour lost office, after which Crossman played no further part in health services reorganisation. But in 1973 he described the Act in its final form as a disaster. He is quoted as saying that the reform aggravated every wrong tendency of the Service in every possible way.[8]

By the mid-1970s it had become increasingly obvious that reorganisation had failed in its intentions and a Royal Commission was set up to examine in detail the problems of the NHS. Its brief was to 'consider in the interests both of the patients and of those who work in the Service the best use and management of the financial and manpower resources'.[9] In a report of nearly 500 pages submitted to the Government in 1979, it reaffirmed principles of the NHS to

> "encourage and assist individuals to remain healthy; provide equality of entitlement to health services; provide a broad range of services of a high standard; provide equality of access to these services; provide a free service at the time of use; satisfy the reasonable expectations of its users; remain a national service responsive to local needs." [10]

It is to the credit of the Commission that it recognised a need to reflect in the provisions of the NHS the differing needs of fit persons to remain healthy from those of the sick for care and treatment. Furthermore, it introduced gradations of care for the latter: 'the self-care which the slightly ill person will exercise which may involve medication and treatment'; 'the care provided by the person's family and by the health and personal social services outside the hospital'; 'the care which can be provided only in hospital or other residential institution'.[11] It accepted that these were not wholly distinct categories and that they would merge into each other: 'A patient should be able to move freely between them as his need for care becomes greater or as he improves . . .. Whatever our needs, administrative barriers should not be created which prevent our being cared for in an effective and convenient way'.[12]

These observations are of particular interest in the context of *Hospital at Home* for two reasons. First, they recognised a need to distinguish, for planning purposes, between the fit and the healthy: raising in an oblique way conflicts of prevention and cure in the roles of GPs. Secondly, they introduced categories of patients defined according to levels and varieties of needs, rather than by medical specialities. Taken together, these two concepts pointed to possibilities of organisational changes which could have provided adequately for patients with high levels and wide varieties of needs, without necessarily institutionalising them. Presumably, the Commission did not want to pursue sensitive issues, on the one hand, concerning relationships between GPs and hospital specialists, on the other, between community health and community social services. Had it done so it might have concluded a need for NHS provision outside hospitals, enabling patients of the above category to receive comprehensive, integrated, domiciliary care, without loss of the treatment benefits they would have received had they been hospitalised.

The Royal Commission put a finger on sources of problems which beset the NHS both before and after its reorganisation. It concluded that what doctors did underlay many of these and did not find arguments put up by the medical profession against salaried GP services convincing, recommending that the option should be introduced – an option which would at least be a step towards integrated patient care. It stressed the importance of integrated health and social services, although it seemed satisfied that in the meantime many problems resulting from existing divisions could be overcome through 'determination on both sides'[13] – an assumption that, to many, would seem to have been unduly optimistic!

The vulnerability of present-day health and social services organisation to demographic variations is illustrated in the Black Report of 1980.[14] Commenting on the findings of the Report, Patrick Jenkin, Secretary of State for Social Services at the time, stated, 'It will come as a disappointment to many that over long periods since the inception of the NHS there is generally little sign of health inequalities in Britain actually diminishing and, in some cases, they may be increasing'.[15] Of course health inequalities stem from many causes (for example, social deprivation, poor housing and employment conditions) which apparently have nothing to do with treatment and care facilities for the sick. But obligation on all members of the medical profession to concern themselves with community facilities for the sick, rather than resort to hospital admissions when problems of home care arise, would result in an awakening of medical awareness of these inequalities. It is to be hoped that this could lead to improvements in health provision currently inconceivable.

The case for a comprehensive secondary care service for the home-bound sick

In the preceding pages I have made a case for the introduction of services which would enable certain patients traditionally hospitalised to remain at home whilst undergoing treatment. Finer definition of the category of patients involved is required before the structure and pattern of services proposed can be usefully described. I have already excluded patients capable of self-care, and those whose needs can be adequately met by help from families, supplemented perhaps by items from primary health and social services. There remains the group which the Royal Commission described as patients requiring care which can be provided only in hospitals or other residential institutions.

Diagnosis, age and treatment needs are not sufficient in themselves to identify persons for whom integrated comprehensive domiciliary care services are required. Most patients are traditionally hospitalised either because they have major treatment needs or because, although treatment needs may be minor, they require high levels of care and support whilst undergoing treatment. Amongst both types of case there are those which might, given parallel facilities, gain greater benefit from home rather than hospital in-patient care. They come potentially from all age groups and, with the exception of cases requiring clinical intervention of kinds impossible outside hospitals, from potentially all diagnostic groups. They might be patients in the terminal stages of illness, or those suffering minor acute medical conditions. But, if of the latter group, major dependency might stem not from the illness itself but, rather, reasons of childhood, advanced age or chronic mental and/or physical incapacity to be found among all age groups.

Thus the potential scope for a secondary home care sickness service is wide. There are, however, certain preliminary requirements for its successful operation. These are based on three assumptions: (1) that the most effective treatment (including its environment) must satisfy not just physical, but also emotional and psychological needs of the patient; (2) that these can best be determined only if the patient is consulted as fully as possible and best satisfied only if a willing party to decisions made (mode of treatment and care must take into full account views and interests of family and others of the patient's entourage likely to be closely affected by arrangements made); (3) that health authorities would not consider widespread introduction of domiciliary alternatives to traditional hospital in-patient care unless they were demonstrably less costly.

Readers already experienced in the care of the dependent sick and the problems of finding satisfactory alternatives to their hospital admission will need no introduction to the types of cases which I have in mind. Others may find it helpful to consider some which I have illustrated below. They come from a wealth of case histories accumulated over my 30 years' experience as a hospital social worker. Cases illustrated relate to patients admitted to a district general hospital in North London during a decade beginning in the mid-1960s and ending in the mid-1970s – a period which covered a time of relative plenty in health and social services resources, and one which spanned the various reorganisation measures designed to make more effective use of these resources. I have omitted types of cases where doctors alone are competent to determine optimum environment of treatment (for example, following major surgery where complications might occur). Such cases would anyway be eligible for secondary domiciliary care if the doctor involved favoured it. In presenting cases of multi-disciplinary needs, where those of nursing and social kinds predominate, I may give readers the impression that 'hospital at home' is a service intended exclusively for the elderly and long-term cases, and, as such, is not a viable alternative to acute hospital medicine. This is emphatically not so, as evidence presented later in this book will confirm.

Case no. 1: Margaret Bailey

Margaret was thirteen when her father lost his leg, eighteen when he died. She describes her experience as follows:

'Following a leg amputation and with a weak heart and blood-clotting, a long stay in hospital for my father seemed inevitable. Unfortunately, he had a great dislike and fear of hospitals which went largely unrecognised by those in charge of his treatment. After three months it was plain to my mother that his very deep depression at remaining there was hindering any hope of recovery and that what he needed was the security and familiarity of his own home. She consequently had him discharged. The importance of this to his well-being was demonstrated by his greatly improved mental outlook and by the fact that, for the first time, he set about coming to terms with his disability. To this day, my mother believes that had he remained in hospital he would never have lived for another five years, the time it took for me to qualify for admission to a teacher-training college, which meant so much to him.

'As there was no real alternative to the hospital care provided, the responsibility for his care rested almost entirely on my mother's shoulders; but instead of being recognised as an important person in the whole process she was frustrated in her attempts to understand and control circumstances and by a lack of communication and sensitivity from those involved. Dad's particular illness did not require continual hospital care, only brief spells, but he needed help with bathing and dressing, special diet, a constant supply of drugs, physiotherapy and, above all, companionship and counselling to help with the many family problems arising from his own and later my mother's illness. We discovered that whilst medical care in long-term illness is usually of a high standard there is a harmful neglect of the patient's mental care and well-being. Most of the time he felt a total sense of humiliation and inadequacy which he had no means of coming to terms with. As well as looking after him my mother went out to work and cared for the interests and problems of two deaf sons and myself, an adolescent daughter. This inevitably placed a great strain on both her relationship with Dad and on her own health.

The treatment he needed meant regular visits to the hospital for physiotherapy and blood tests with their attendant problems of waiting, sometimes for hours, for transport, and the whole impersonality of hospital treatment, which would leave Dad exhausted and nervous for days on end. Our greatest concern was that, if for any reason Mum became unable to cope, Dad would have to be re-admitted to hospital as he simply could not manage without a great deal of help. This led to a situation where we would not call in the doctor at times when he was needed; in my mother's case, she refused to enter hospital for tests, fearing she would have to stay in for a hysterectomy. Finally she became so ill that this could no longer be avoided, and it was discovered that she had advanced cancer of the cervix. Had a well organised system of home care at the level Dad needed been available, her fears about what would have become of him could have been allayed to enable her to have treatment much earlier.

'For the next two years she spent more time in hospital than out. When she was at home she needed constant rest but did not get it, as she attempted to resume her former role of caring for my father. He suffered deeply from guilt at this situation and both of them felt isolated by each other's illness. At this time the only aid we were offered was a home help for two hours twice a week, a totally inadequate measure given the circumstances. As my mother was not expected to live much longer, I was told by my general practitioner not to worry as my dad would then be permanently hospitalised and my one brother still at home placed in a hostel. Whether or not this situation could ever have arisen I had no way of knowing at the time and the only effect it had was to make me take on my mum's role of protecting what was left of the family from further break-up. Believing that any sign that we could not cope would lead to hospital for my dad, we concealed major problems and refused to go for help when it was badly needed. Very often he needed oxygen to combat his shortness of breath but we feared that to ask for this would mean hospital so we kept quiet. Many times he missed his much-needed physiotherapy treatment because he was too ill to face the journey. It was left to relatives and kindly neighbours to help him bath as this was one job his pride would not let me do.

'Dad died five years after his amputation, not many months after Mum returned home from hospital. For the last two years of his life they had seen little of one another and only then under very difficult circumstances. In the last few days of his life he pleaded with us not to allow him to be put into hospital but because of his great pain and incontinence we had no alternative, given my mother's still precarious state of health. I made the decision to call the doctor who immediately had him admitted and we were told that he would not return. We were all deeply distressed by my action and I felt profoundly guilty. The only treatment he received on this final occasion was oxygen, pain-killing drugs and a catheter, all of which could have been administered in his own home had we only had extra support to help us in our own efforts to hold things together and to cope with the extra work involved. The memory which remains strongest to us about the last days of his life is the enormous distress at what he regarded as the final indignity of ending his life in a hospital bed.'

Case no. 2: Thomas Bridges

Thomas Bridges was forty. He had apparently been a fit man until the day he collapsed at work following a cerebral haemorrhage. His wife worked part-time and there were two children aged eight and six years. Following a prolonged stay in hospital, which meant he lost his job, he was eventually discharged from hospital to the care of his wife, who gave up work to look after him. A few months later he had a second stroke and was re-admitted to hospital. This time he lost the use of an arm and a leg and became incontinent, confused and unable to speak clearly. As he was depressed and frustrated in hospital his wife decided to look after him at home. The district nurses, home help service, Red Cross and other voluntary bodies gave as much help as they could and twice a week Mr Bridges was taken by ambulance to the hospital physiotherapy department.

Almost every day, however, there was some sort of misunderstanding which caused friction and made Mrs Bridges feel uncomfortable. Sometimes the district nurse did not arrive until she had managed to wash her husband and change his bed-linen on her own. Sometimes the ambulance was delayed by several hours and sometimes it came before she and the nurse had managed to get her husband ready. If she decided to leave the shopping until the home help came, the home help might not arrive at all; if she set to and did all the housework, the home help would arrive, gaining the impression that her services were not needed. Sometimes several helpers would all call at the same time – the Red Cross lady, the nurse, the home help and the social worker – and it would look as if Mrs Bridges was being excessively demanding. At other times no one would call throughout the day and the children would come home from school to a harassed mother and the house in turmoil.

Seemingly it would have been better for the family in this case if Mr Bridges had remained in hospital. Such was my own view at the time. Apart from the disruption his presence at home must have caused for the family, hardly a week went by without protest from the primary care services that his case was too much of a strain for them, leading to the neglect of other needy cases. But Mrs Bridges was an unusual woman. She was intensely religious, believing that the task of caring for her husband was heaven-sent. She cared deeply that her children should not suffer deprivation resulting from the heavy demands placed upon her by her husband. Her energy and patience were apparently inexhaustible. She would not accept that, in view of the uncertain future for herself and her children, she might be wise to continue in her part-time work and allow her husband to be looked after in hospital.

In the event, inevitably, the mental and physical strains of trying to cope without the outside support so desperately needed were too much for her. She became depressed and unhappy at what she felt to be her own failure. Her mental breakdown led to the permanent hospital admission of her husband, and worse, her children had to be taken into the care of the local authority.

Case no. 3: Rosina Garrett

Mrs Garrett, a nursing sister, was looking forward to her retirement when it was found that she had advanced cancer of the breast. Following an unsuccessful operation, her husband was advised that her life expectation might be around six months. As it happened she survived for a further two years, but for much of that time she was bedridden and in considerable pain. Her deepest fear was that she might have to end her days in hospital. She had a comfortable home, supportive family, and many good friends, all of whom were willing to work together towards her home care. There were times during the day, however, when none of them was able to be with her for reasons of work or family commitment. Being a member of the nursing sisterhood, Mrs Garrett received more frequent attention from district nurses than would have otherwise been likely. This, and the home help arranged for her, might have proved adequate to cover the absence of family and friends, had it been possible to draw up a rota of attendance. But no one could be certain when either nurse or home help would call; and, although Mrs Garrett's husband and sons worked closed to home and had helpful employers who would have been happy to vary their hours to enable such a rota, this proved impracticable. When her condition deteriorated and she required constant attention day and night, night nurses attended her several times a week to enable the family to get some sleep. In view of the cost, however, the health authority was unable to finance this beyond a few weeks.

Had Mrs Garrett survived only the six months originally predicted by her doctors she might have been enabled to stay at home until her death. But the impossibility of making satisfactory plans for this over an indefinite period proved too much for her family and the primary care services responsible. She therefore had to be admitted to hospital where she spent several unhappy months, her family distressed and feeling guilty at having allowed this to happen.

Case no 4: Hugh Jenkins

When Hugh was twelve years old he was run over by a car and admitted to the intensive care unit of the hospital where I worked at the time. He was critically injured and the doctors were not optimistic about his prospects of regaining consciousness. For many weeks members of his large family kept constant vigil over him. When he finally came around, it was feared that brain damage would be permanent, apart from which broken bones and other serious injuries left his life in the balance for some months.

Against medical expectations Hugh's condition steadily improved until he was fit to leave the intensive care unit for the children's ward. But his injuries and impaired mental state, together with the problems inherent in trying to contain a twelve-year-old in a ward of younger sick children made necessary his transfer to an adult unit. This arrangement was equally unsatisfactory, but for different reasons. Some patients in the adult ward had suffered heart attacks, others chest diseases and strokes; some were in the advanced stages of senility. The unit was not equipped to meet the needs of a child, and staff had niether the time nor the understanding to meet Hugh's needs. He became progressively more noisy and disruptive and a constant source of worry both to staff and to the other patients. He had to wear a padded helmet to protect him from further injury on his frequent falls. Sometimes he escaped the ward and would be found in the street or the hospital grounds, trying to find his way home.

Hugh's parents wanted to look after him at home: but they could not cope with more than the occasional weekend when the older children were around and able to help with the younger ones. When his condition in hospital began to deteriorate, however, they decided that, regardless of the problems, they must accept responsibility for his discharge. The hospital doctors were not happy with the arrangement, but, along with other hospital staff, were relieved by his parents' decision. The GP in the case was deeply concerned that adequate community help would not be available, but nevertheless accepted that, regardless of the dangers, home care could not be so damaging to Hugh's interests as was hospital in the circumstances.

Meanwhile, Hugh continued to need physio-, occupational and speech therapy – facilities available in the area only through the hospital sector and on hospital premises. This involved hospital visits by ambulance three times a week. In addition the district nurse was required to make daily visits – Hugh was still incontinent and his injuries had not fully healed. On occasions Mrs Jenkins had to be absent from home when no other member of the family could be present to keep an eye on him (for example, when shopping or keeping a school appointment). She did not require help with her housework but the support of some motherly person who understood her son's needs would have been invaluable at these times.

Lack of integrated and co-ordinated hospital and community health and social services made impossible in Hugh's case a routine which would have enabled him to live at home whilst gaining maximum benefit from hospital facilities. Had circumstances been different he might have made a faster and more complete recovery than that which took place.

Doctors variously estimate that at a given time around 30 per cent of patients in Britain are unnecessarily hospitalised. Such estimations are, however, meaningless. Any patient whose home environment inhibits recovery requires either modifications to that environment remedying the situation or removal to somewhere more suitable – usually a hospital. Apparently, modifications traditionally in the form of help and support from health or social service authorities have not appreciably reduced levels of hospital admissions over the years: despite the fact that during the past decade many areas have set up home care schemes specifically designed to avoid hospital admissions or to facilitate early discharge.

Where major dependency on others is involved, patient options in favour of home care, tempered with agreement from other responsible members of the patient's household, are essential in the interests both of the latter and of the health authority involved. This is because, however great its commitment, no authority can entirely relieve the family of ultimate patient responsibility, save by a hospital admission. In the absence of patient choice and family agreement there are many ways in which the presence of domiciliary alternatives to hospital admission might be mis-used by professionals under pressure to conserve hospital beds.

We do not know what percentage of patients traditionally hospitalised under the NHS would, given the chance, opt for home care alternatives such as described in the pages which follow. But overseas experiment suggests that there are sufficient numbers to warrant its introduction as a permanent part of hospital services of any developed health system – ranging from private, through insurance-backed, to socialised and nationalised services.

References

(1) Abel-Smith, B., *The Hospitals 1800–1948*, Heinemann, London, 1964, p. 454; Honigsbaum, F., *The Division in British Medicine*, Kogan Page, London, 1979, p. 217.
(2) Honigsbaum, *op. cit.*, p. 144.
(3) *Ibid.*, p. 175.

(4) Cang, S., and Clarke, F., 'Home care of the sick – an emerging general analysis based on schemes in France', *Community Health*, 1978, **9** (3), 167–71.

(5) *Report of the Committee on Local Authority and Allied Personal Social Services* (Chairman: F. Seebohm), Cmmd 3603, HMSO, London, 1968.

(6) *Local Authority Social Services Act 1970*, HMSO, London, 1970, chapter 42.

(7) *Royal Commission on the National Health Service Report* (Chairman: Sir Alec Merrison), HMSO, London, 1979.

(8) *Social Worker*, 26 July 1973.

(9) Royal Commission's Report, *op. cit.*, para 1.1.

(10) *Ibid.*, para 2.6.

(11) *Ibid.*, p. 39.

(12) *Ibid.*, p. 39.

(13) *Ibid.*, para 22.57.

(14) *Inequalities in Health: Report of a Research Working Group* (Chairman: Sir Douglas Black), DHSS, London, 1980.

(15) *Ibid.*, Foreword.

4 Overseas experiments in the home care of the sick

The NHS is presently under critical scrutiny both from its advocates and its adversaries. A powerful section of the medical profession has declared itself in favour of private medicine, while the Government of the day has expressed interest in insurance-backed health schemes which, if introduced in Britain, could destroy concepts of an egalitarian service universally free at the time of need. It is therefore crucial that we should consider whether there is anything which can be usefully learned from overseas health experience and introduced to the NHS without undermining concepts which have proved to be of inestimable benefit to the British people over nearly four decades.

Hospital social workers are particularly aware of inequalities in health provision because they are in daily contact with patients and their families who suffer them most. So, perhaps it is not surprising that someone like myself, who has witnessed first hand the sufferings and indignities caused by means testing of pre-NHS days, should view with concern the possibility of their return. At the same time I am acutely aware that the NHS has failed to resolve problems of unwanted and harmful institutionalisation, the most dreaded form of Poor Law provision of earlier days.

It was at the time of searching debate about reorganisation proposals of the early 1970s that I first heard of a hospital-based home care service in France called 'hospitalisation à domicile' (HAD). I discovered that 'l'Assistance Publique', the public authority responsible for hospital services of the Paris region, had established a highly successful extramural service to which patients already occupying general hospital beds could, if they wished, apply for 'admission'. Under the scheme their hospital-prescribed treatments would be continued in their home environments by specialists working in liaison with family doctors. I was told that the arrangement required agreement of clinical responsibility between specialist and GP before transfer from hospital bed to home care under HAD could take place; that the arrangement included agreement of the specialist to see the patient regularly once a fortnight and of the GP to visit the patient at home regularly twice a week; that HAD itself undertook all other responsibilities for patient well-being in much the same way as do hospitals; that the scheme co-ordinated its activities with those of hospital doctor and GP and the willing and able contribution of the patient's family and other entourage.

In 1972, enabled by a grant from the Council of Europe, I spent a month with l'Assistance Publique observing HAD in operation and studying the system under which it operates. In the following year I spent a month at the Ecôle Nationale de la Santé Publique (National School of Public Health) in Rennes to gain deeper knowledge of French health and social services: from whence I learned of other HAD schemes in France and also of hospital-based home care services operating on similar lines in other parts of the world.

In France I found widespread admiration for the NHS but little apparent desire for its emulation. Seemingly, the French were reasonably satisfied with their own system. I found the paperwork of the latter tiresome and complicated but, by and large, standards and varieties of its provisions seemed roughly comparable to those of the NHS. In both there is an obvious lack of adequate provision for the care of the dependent sick at home through traditional services; but, apparently, in France there are no organisational obstacles of a kind inherent in the NHS to experiment outside traditional patterns, bringing within a common structure the activities of family doctors and hospital consultants.

An article reporting my findings of the Paris experiment, published in 1973,[1] aroused widespread and enthusiastic interest in this country amongst health professionals and administrators, academics, and, most significantly, from lay persons and groups, usually more concerned with the benevolent aspects of patient care than notions of structure and organisation. The article led to radio and television broadcasts and a steady flow of requests to speak at meetings, seminars and conferences, to describe more fully the French experience of 'hospital at home'.

In 1977, thanks to a grant from the Nuffield Foundation, I was enabled, together with Stephen Cang, a member of the Health Service Organisation Research Unit of Brunel University, to spend some weeks in France examining HAD concepts and operations in greater depth than had hitherto been possible. At the time of our visit, the various separate schemes which, in the main, had simulated the Paris experience were in the process of formulating basic aims and principles of organisation and operation through a national federation established in 1974 (La Fédération Nationale des Etablissements d'Hospitalisation à Domicile). These joint study visits enabled analysis of the French schemes from which we concluded that there existed problems of ideological significance in the development of domiciliary patient care, inhibiting to both French and British health systems. However, we also concluded that a facility open to the French people had been demonstrated which to date was not available under the NHS.

I have described the French experience of *hospitalisation à domicile* in detail in chapter 5. In chapter 6 I have described some home care projects introduced to the NHS in recent years with aims similar to those of the French schemes, but lacking the clear-cut organisation of the latter. First, however, a brief survey of hospital-based home care experiments in various other developed countries overseas suggests the extent of global interest in seeking alternatives to hospital admission. It also confirms obstacles to providing combinations of general and specialist care (sometimes as essential to patients at home as in hospital) common to many health systems based on Western European medicine.

A global sketch of health care alternatives

A characteristic of all developed countries is the existence of forms of social security which provide and maintain minimum standards of health and social care for individual citizens. These standards are recognised to be important to the conditions of the public at large. On this basis nearly all countries of the world now provide some forms of statutory health and social services which are developed as wealth increases and standards rise.

The existence of health and social provision does not seem to be contingent upon ideology or economic considerations (although the *nature* and *structure* of such provision may be). Socialist countries aim to provide comprehensive care as the right of every citizen; but many private enterprise countries which are highly industrialised and which have long traditions of social awareness now practice policies which, however complex in their operation, are virtually comprehensive in effect. Arrangements for state care vary from that which is directly organised by statutory agencies to that which is chanelled through private agencies. In some countries, for example in France, private health provision flourishes alongside that of the state to the point where the two systems can provide an integrated pattern of comprehensive care. In others, for example in the UK, the 'partnership' between the two sectors is uneasy and disparities between services provided through the public and the private sectors persist.

In global terms four main types of health provision may be distinguished:

(1) In advanced market economics, including those of the EEC and the non-aligned countries which operate similar systems (for example, Sweden, Australia, Canada), standards rise as wealth increases, but the private sector advances alongside, and frequently ahead of, the public sector.

(2) In centrally planned economies all services are state-run; as living standards rise so too does the overall level of health and social welfare provision.

(3) In the oil-based economies such as apply in the Arab states, where traditionally all properties (including women) are privately owned, medicine is also private, but the state intervenes where necessary towards the maintenance of minimum acceptable standards;

(4) Third World countries, which still have to contend with massive problems of famine and disease, tend towards broad-based programmes of state medicine, although traditional practices continue alongside attempts to modernise the approach.

In industrially advanced countries, whether socialist or market economies, minimum provisions are not dissimilar. Even in the USA free medical care for essential treatment is available to those who are unable to pay for it, *if* the particular medical condition is considered to be socially unacceptable.

Britain has made a name for herself as leader in health care provision largely because she was the first country to introduce a nationalised health service. Many other countries now, however, appear to have as high or higher levels of provision, through structures and patterns of development radically different from those which apply in Britain (see table 4.1).

Table 4.1   Levels of health care provision in European countries in 1978.

	Health cost (£ per head)	Percentage of gross domestic product spent on health (%)	Gross domestic product (£ per head)	Practising doctors per 100 000 people	Hospital beds per 1000 people
West Germany	425	7.8	5435	215	11.8
Netherlands	413	8.4	4890	171	12.3
Denmark	412	7.2	5710	200	8.0
Belgium	300	6.0	5000	225	9.1
Luxembourg	296	5.8	5110	163	12.9
France	290	6.3	4620	172	11.5
United Kingdom	159	5.5	2885	150	8.1
Ireland	126	6.6	1920	118	10.1
Italy	109	4.6	2390	245	9.9
EEC	261	6.6	3970	197	10.3

Source: Demographic and Statistical Department of the European Commission and health departments of the nine members of the EEC[2]

Disregarding other factors, however, a number of overseas countries operate hospital-based domiciliary care schemes which appear to offer facilities more comprehensive and better organised than are the primary care services of the UK, which have difficulty in defining both their responsibilities and methods of meeting them.

Home care schemes in the United States of America

In 1948, Dr E. M. Bluestone, Director of the Montefiore Hospital, New York, decided to extend his hospital service to enable patients who wished it to be looked after in their own homes. He accordingly introduced a demonstration project of combined hospital–home organisation to add an extramural dimension to traditional intramural hospital services. The project was to become an inspiration and guide for similar schemes throughout the world. (Dr Bluestone died at the age of 87 in 1979, a year in which he recorded appreciation that his pioneering contribution to the home care of the sick should have been acknowledged in the author's attempt to bring 'hospital at home' to the UK.[3])

Bluestone maintained that those responsible should think twice before removing any patients from home surroundings, whether for the overtly apparent benefit of the patient or that of the medical attendant. He considered that, in the first place, the possibilities of continued home care under subsidised conditions should be investigated – transfer to hospital, he said, should never be a simple matter of expedience but of inescapable necessity.[3]

Bluestone recommended that, as soon as a working diagnosis had been made, the desirable place of treatment should be considered jointly by physician and social worker; the purpose being to get a combined judgement on the best place for the patient under all the circumstances of the illness. Where the social worker reported an inadequate home, efforts should be made to make it adequate by one kind of subsidy or another. Three valid reasons for an essential hospital admission were, he argued: the need for major surgery; the need for comprehensive investigation and treatment with intensive use of hospital laboratories, under specialised observation and control; the need for heavy non-portable equipment. Where these reasons did not prevail he considered the home (or substitute home) to be the preferred environment of treatment, with the patients under the care of the family doctor and the hospital standing by.

American hospitals as they are known today had come into being less than two centuries before, in response to the increasing number of diagnostic and therapeutic inventions and discoveries which were being employed in the treatment of the sick. They were built on the assumption that more seriously sick patients could not be left at home. Much later, in an effort to bridge the gap between medical provision and the unmet social needs of patients, medical-social services were introduced into these hospitals, but then only to deal with so-called 'charity cases'. In the development of hospital-based home care programmes, Dr Bluestone foresaw the potential for developing medical social services amongst all patients, at home and in hospital.[4]

This extramural dimension to the traditional hospital services at Montefiore came into being at a time when medical and social sciences were converging, bringing the needs of the patient into stereoscopic view. The services of 'Home Care', as the scheme is called, made it possible and eminently practicable to reconsider the organisation and delivery of medical care, so as to make it more effective, more comprehensive and more continuous than ever before. 'Home Care' bridged the gap, 'sometimes a yawning chasm', said Bluestone, between hospital and home.[5]

Twenty-five years later he felt confident in claiming that his project had stood the test of thorough experimentation so that its principles might be easily applied wherever there was a need. By this time the experiment at Montefiore Hospital no longer stood alone, because numerous schemes based on his ideas had been introduced throughout the world and had themselves proved to be of inestimable value both to those who worked in them and to the patients who benefited from them.

Medical services in the USA are private and consequently are discriminatory in their application. Bluestone felt justified in his claim that his scheme helped to equalise the distribution of hospital resources to wherever they were most needed. Subsidising the patient to enable care to take place at home, he claimed, reduced the incidence and degree of their exclusion from medical care and treatment.

But his interest was not confined to medical intervention alone. His scheme included provision for those whose treatment needs were limited. He referred to arbitrary classification such as 'acute' and 'chronic' as being 'semantic impediments to humane service which too often become confused with terms that have very different meanings: for example, "convalescent", "aged", "custodial", ... Each of these distinct entities', he said, 'has its corresponding resource within an integrated hospital-home pattern of medical care.'[6] He questioned prognosis in terms of curability, pointing out that 'curable' means we have the required facilities, knowledge and skills to deal with the condition in a responsive patient. 'Incurable' means that we do not have these requirements, or the sustained interest in discovering the means to make the condition curable. 'It is', he said, 'from the incurable that we can still hope for cures, not from the curable who have already benefited from such interest.'[7] Bluestone claimed that no other facility has ever been established that can do the job of effecting cure better than a hospital. Since incurability so often goes hand in hand with impoverishment, traditional sources of financial and material relief must be absorbed into the pattern of care for the home-bound patient, just as when associated with the need for food and shelter alone; and for this to be done the traditional resources of the hospital had to be mobilised to reach people in their own homes. 'All these threads', he said, referring to the many aspects in which his 'Home Care' service has advantages over traditional hospital care, 'can now be woven into a responsible pattern of medical organisation which will leave no sick person out in the cold, whether acutely or chronically ill, ambulatory or bedfast, rich or poor, young or old, mentally or physically sick.'[8]

Schemes inspired by the pioneering efforts of Dr Bluestone have proliferated in the United States since 1948. For example, Los Angeles County–University of Southern California Medical Center (LAC-USC) – a large urban hospital – has found that many modern problems of health care can be resolved by the reintroduction of house-calls by hospital doctors under a scheme sometimes described as a 'hospital without walls'.[7] Here physicians are available seven days a week, 24 hours a day, to follow through the same patients for as long as they remain the responsibility of the project. The scheme claims particular success in the care of patients suffering a number of different illnesses which may be associated with and affected by each other.[10]

In 1966, in Portland, Oregan, the Kaiser–Permanente Medical Care system introduced into its home care provisions a programme of extended hospital facilities under a comprehensive prepayment plan.[11] This programme was designed to produce data to evaluate legislative proposals for financing a similar service for the majority of the United States population dependent on insurance reimbursement for their health care. Of particular interest to this book is the programme's concept of 'home health aides' (also known as *aides-soignantes* – in France, home care assistants, and patients' aides) whose services were enlisted following appropriate training to assume an increasing share of nursing, social work and physiotherapy duties, under close professional supervision. The project at first experienced considerable resistance to the idea from the professionals involved, resistance which has been softened but not entirely overcome as the value of these home health aides has been realised.

Commenting on the rights of patients to be looked after in their own homes where medically feasible, an article on the San Fransisco Home Health Service published in 1975[12] suggests that a selection and combination of services to meet the needs of a patient at any given time must be capable of prompt adjustment and change in kind, intensity and duration, focused on the individual rather than on groups whose needs may be disparate. In this way they provide for economies in utilisation of both professional and paraprofessional staff, making therapeutic use of the environment and eliminating necessity for adjustment to an environment which may not accord with the life-style of the individual. They thus have the potential to preserve pre-existing relationships, enhancing participation in normal community life and encouraging maximum utilisation of family, friends and community services. They make extensive use of well trained, supervised paraprofessionals, who increase the capacities of professional staffs, providing patients with personalised continuity of contact and relationship with those responsible for care services.[13]

Numerous American states now run hospital-based home care schemes on the lines described above. But since each state determines its own policy, an overall assessment of domiciliary patient care in the USA is impossible. However, in 1973 the Board to Trustees of the American Hospitals Association issued a policy statement urging full support and utilisation of home health care services in the interests of both patients and hospitals. This was endorsed by the National League of Nursing and the

National Association of Home Health agencies. The American Medical Association has now formally accepted the statement's principles.[14]

When the idea of home care as an alternative to hospitalisation was first introduced in America it seemed that obstacles to its realisation were ideological, psychological and financial. Now that experiment has proved its benefits and relative economies of cost, other objections to the idea appear to inhibit its spread: 'not within the hospital's province to send teams into patient' homes', said one hospital administrator; 'In view of an 80 % bed occupancy rate it would be self-defeating to set up a home-care program which will syphon off more patients', said another; and 'I am running a deficit now and can't add to it by taking on a home-care service', said a third.[15] Such comments are representative of many expressed throughout countries whose services are designed and run to satisfy professional and administrative interests even, sometimes, at the expense of their sick citizens.

Canada

Some Canadian provinces have developed their health services well beyond minimum requirements laid down and in part financed by the Federal Government.[16] In 1971 the latter approved in principle the setting up of special projects making available, free of charge, services necessary to enable the early discharge of hospital patients who might thereby be effectively looked after at home. The provision covers nursing and medical attention, drugs, equipment, supplies, transportation, laboratory services, home-makers, meals on wheels and other social support services, enabling socially advanced provinces such as British Columbia, Edmonton, Manitoba and Quebec to add radically to imaginative home care programmes, some of which have been in practice for up to 30 years. [17] In addition to schemes providing alternatives to general hospital admission, these include special services for patient groups such as children and the terminally ill.

Australia

In 1979 the Australian Commonwealth Department of Health published its findings on relative home care, nursing home and hospital costs.[18] These confirmed earlier studies made in Britain and the USA, concluding that, depending on methods of assessment used, between 10 and 33 per cent of patients in acute hospitals could have been effectively treated in less expensive institutions or at home.[19] As the Australian study points out, cost analysis comparisons between widely differing health systems and demographic conditions are liable to inaccuracies and inconsistencies. Even within Australia there are wide variations in health facilities provided by its federated states, so that generalisations throughout the Commonwealth are of necessity broad. From the experience of pioneering schemes set up in various parts of that country to remedy problems in inadequate domiciliary care for the sick, however, we do know that Australia shares with countries such as the UK, France, Canada and the USA concern about the failure of traditional health services to make adequate provision for patient care outside their hospitals.

General practice in Australia is almost entirely paid for on a 'fee for service' basis, backed largely by non-profit-making insurance provision. Virtually the only hospital beds to which GPs have access are in the private sector. Specialists are free to prescribe for patients in their own homes, although the practice is not common.

Until the 1970s virtually the only organised services able to help the sick in their own homes were those of district nurses and meals on wheels. In 1971, in Adelaide, South Australia, a small-scale experiment was pioneered by the Department of Physical Medicine of Queen Elizabeth district hospital. It grew rapidly, soon covering a population of 280 000. Within three years three similar schemes were opened to cover the whole of the metropolitan area, followed by 14 others in the surrounding country districts.[20] The experiment is known as the Western Domiciliary Care Service. It was enabled following an offer from the Australian Minister of Health, in 1969, of statutory financing on a dollar-for-dollar basis, as an incentive to set up facilities for comprehensive domiciliary care.[21]

Of particular interest to students of home care in Britain is the means found by the Western Domiciliary Care Service of drawing into a hospital-based scheme traditional district nursing services of the area. This was achieved by the basing of a district nursing supervisor at the care centre to minimise problems of liaison and other professional relationships. Paramedical aides, domiciliary helpers and home helps, responsible for all non-nursing duties involving 'looking-after' the patient and ensuring a satisfactory environment of care, however, remain the responsibility of the Service itself, usually under the supervision of its paramedical and social workers, not nurses employed by local district nursing services.

The need to rely on professional nursing help from outside the Care Service does create problems of liaison and co-ordination of work which have proved difficult to overcome. Despite enormous benefits of patient interest claimed over those of traditional community care arrangements for the dependent sick in Australia, the Western Domiciliary Care Service acknowledges ideological and practical difficulties in determining where to draw the line between primary care activities and its own hospital-based intervention.

The Co-ordinated Care Scheme at Mount Royal Hospital in Melbourne, Victoria, has experienced similar problems. The Medical Director of this scheme for the elderly, set up in 1974, stresses the crucial importance of such a service being 'visible' to the population to whom it applies. Towards this end leaflets and other publicity are freely circulated in the tongues of Greek, German, Latvian, Maltese and Turkish minority groups as well as in English.[22]

Throughout Australia there is now a trend towards diversified health care programmes, bringing together hospital- and community-based services. These are usually aimed at meeting the needs of the elderly and disabled, as can be seen from a comprehensive list of projects compiled in the late 1970s.[23] But schemes like the Western Domiciliary Care Service and (more lately) the Southern Domiciliary Care Service in South Adelaide are now being emulated on an ever widening scale, indicating Australian recognition of the need to base patient services on individual levels and varieties of need rather than on group categorisation by age and medical diagnosis alone.

New Zealand

Under its National Health Service, the health of the people of New Zealand is the responsibility of a partnership of central and local government similar to that which applies in the UK. For many years prior to the introduction of extramural activities into the programme of the Auckland Hospital Board in 1960, it had been widely accepted that district hospitals had responsibilities to provide certain services to patients in their own homes and that hospitals gained from this to the extent that better use could thereby be made of hospital beds. Different boards interpreted their responsibilities in different ways, however, and it was not until the New Zealand Board of Health made official recommendations on the proper scope and future development of hospital extramural services that individual hospitals were able to develop plans of their own based on these and local needs and possibilities.[24]

The Auckland Extramural Hospital is statutorily obliged to limit its facilities to *bona fide* patients only – that is, to people requiring medical, surgical or nursing care and treatment, who traditionally would expect to be admitted to an institution for these services. It was from the effort to co-ordinate under one direction activities of a domiciliary and out-patient nature and the contribution of other agencies, voluntary societies and groups, that the concept of an extramural hospital developed. The idea was to provide total programmes of care and treatment to points where specialised knowledge and equipment available only in hospitals was required.

In its first phase, the Extramural Hospital relied on co-ordinated activities alone and for this period its growth and effectiveness was limited. But when, in 1968, a headquarters was created and the various services involved were brought together under one roof, the scheme was immediately able to expand and develop as a fully integrated service. Staff from all disciplines got to know each other, co-ordinating their activities simply and naturally and without the time-wasting procedures hitherto involved in bringing them together. In 1976 the Medical Superintendent of the Auckland Hospital Board reported an estimated halving of the times many patients were having to spend in hospital as a result of Extramural Hospital operation. He quoted a recent research finding in Wellington, New Zealand, that 39.6 per cent of patients in hospital at any one time were being given treatment no different from that being provided in the homes of the sick in the area, confirming his own estimate of at least 30 per cent who could be equally well looked after at home as in hospital.[25]

Other home care schemes

No useful purpose would be served in this book by mentioning all other overseas home care initiatives which have been brought to my notice in the course of research. It may be that there are others more impressive, in countries where language barriers make it difficult to gain accurate information, than those I have mentioned. For example, hospital at home schemes have been introduced in Helsinki Municipal Hospital, Finland, in 1954,[29] and in the Soviet Union (Leningrad, Moscow and Minsk) in the early 1960s.[30] Alternatively, it may be that the development of home care in preference to that of institutions is but a part of modern social development unhampered by traditions of centuries, for example as in Israel, where, following the Yom Kippur War of 1973, the Kupat Holim (Israel's major national health insurance organisation) set up its first Home Care Unit based on the out-patient and community care services in the Rishon Le Zion area of Tel Aviv.[31]

Conclusions

My purpose in mentioning this overseas experience is to convey to readers the global extent of interest in seeking alternatives to medically unnecessary and unwanted hospital admissions which are both humane and economic. It might well be that economic considerations in practice over-ride those of particular patient benefit. Nevertheless, time and again, we are brought back by the early pioneers of structured home care to the fundamental importance of considering first and foremost the circumstances and aspirations of individual patients and their families.

British, American and Australian research calculations suggest that between 10 and 30 per cent of traditionally hospitalised patients could be well provided for either at home or in institutions cheaper to run than general hospitals. Whatever the percentages, however, it seems that organisational and professional obstacles to looking after the sick at home are greater than those of funding and resources.

In determining the precise nature of provision required for heavily dependent patients at home in the UK, we should take note of the view widely held overseas that such patients should be the responsibility of the hospital sectors of the various health systems concerned: the reason being that GPs alone cannot command either the resources or specialist skills which might be as essential in cases of major illness in the home as in hospital. Some overseas countries have apparently been able to develop schemes integrating specialist and GP care for the sick at home because demarcations between these two professional groups are not so rigid as in the UK (many GPs overseas also hold hospital appointments in some specialism or another). Ultimately, however, all patients, whatever their country of origin, are obliged to accept environments of treatment chosen by their doctors. Only in this way can a delicate balance of medical interests be maintained. Wherever such interests are favoured by hospital-orientated medicine, opportunities for patients to be treated in their preferred environment of the home are certain to be limited. This may be the reason why, although successful, 'hospital at home' schemes overseas have remained small in size and number. Where, as under the NHS, organisation reinforces notions of a divided medical profession, prospects for the development of home care alternatives to general hospital admission are apparently poorer than, for example, in France, where liberal medicine enables more diversified patient care.

A survey in chapter 6 of home care initiatives in Britain over the past decade illustrates my point. But, first, a more detailed description of *hospitalisation à domicile* in France will, I hope, enable readers to judge for themselves features of the latter which might add to the benefits of nationalised health care in this country.

References and notes

(1) Clarke, F., 'Hospital at home', *Health and Social Services Journal*, 9 June 1973, 1311–2.

(2) Shrank, A., 'The pounds, francs and marks of health care and why Britain is so far down the league table', *The Times*, 29 October 1980.

(3) Letter to the author from John Dodd, overseas correspondent of the British Hospitals Contributory Schemes Association, 1979.

(4) Bluestone, E. M., 'The contribution of the hospital to the sick man's home', *World Hospitals*, 1974, **10** (2), 92–4. For further information on the Montefiore Hospital Home Care Service, see also the following: *Procedure Manual for Home Care*, revised edition, Montefiore Hospital and Medical Center, New York, 1973; Rossman, I., 'The Montefiore Hospital after-care program', *Nursing Outlook*, 1974, **22** (5), 325–8; Rossman, I., *et al.*, 'Alternatives to institutional care', *Bulletin of the New York Academy of Medicine*, 1973, **49** (12), 1084–92; Rossman, I., *et al.*, 'Total rehabilitation in a home care setting', *New York State Journal of Medicine*, 1962, **62** (8), 1215–9.

(5) Bluestone, *op. cit.*

(6) *Ibid.*

(7) *Ibid.*

(8) *Ibid.*

(9) Yeager, R., 'Hospital treats patients at home', *Modern Health Care*, 1975, **4** (4), 29–32.

(10) *Ibid.*

(11) Arnold, V., *et al.*, *Home Care and Extended Care in a Comprehensive Prepayment Plan*, Kaiser-Permanente Medical Care System, Portland, Ore., undated.

(12) *Home Maker Home Health Aide Services Inc. Basic National Standards – A Giant Step towards Quality Care*, Home Health Aide Services Inc., New York, undated.

(13) *Ibid.*

(14) Richter, L., and Gonnerman, A., 'Home health services and hospitals – an American health authority survey', *Hospitals*,

Journal of the American Hospitals Association, 1974, **48** (1), 113–6; Trager, B., 'Providing the right to stay at home', *Hospitals, Journal of the American Hospitals Association*, 1975, **49** (20), 93–8.

(15) Rossman, I., 'The after-care project: a viable alternative to home care', *Medical Care*, 1974, **11** (6), 235.

(16) *Health and Welfare in Canada: Part I. Health Services*, revised edition, Reference Papers No. 92, Information Division, Department of External Affairs, Ottawa, 1975.

(17) Crane, L. M., 'Home care programs in BC', *Hospital Administration in Canada*, 1975, **17** (10), 28–31; Rioux, C., 'Health and social services under the same roof', *The Canadian Nurse*, 1975, **71** (5), 24–6; Address by E. Shapiro (Assistant Professor, Dept of Social and Preventive Medicine, Faculty of Medicine, University of Manitoba) to the National Seminar on Home Care, as recorded in the Canadian Dept. of National Health and Welfare, Summary and Proceedings of National Seminar on Home Care, Ottawa, April 13–15, 1981; Richardson, B. G., 'Home care programs in Canada: A health management forum, **2** (4), Winter 1981 review, 57–64.

(18) *Relative Costs of Home Care and Nursing Home and Hospital Care in Australia*, Commonwealth Department of Health Monograph Series No. 10, Commonwealth Department of Health, Canberra, 1979.

(19) *Ibid.*, p. 92.

(20) Burnell, A. W., 'The Western Domiciliary Care Service', unpublished paper, Queen Elizabeth Hospital, Adelaide, undated; Burnell, S. F., 'Where do we draw the line?' unpublished paper, Queen Elizabeth Hospital, Adelaide, undated; Burnell, S. F., 'Multipurpose aides for domiciliary care', unpublished paper, Queen Elizabeth Hospital, Adelaide, undated; Munday, C. G., 'Development of domiciliary services in South Australia with special reference to the Western Domiciliary Care Service', unpublished paper, Queen Elizabeth Hospital, Adelaide, undated

(21) Munday, *op. cit.*

(22) Russell, B., 'Co-ordinated care scheme', *Age Concern Today*, Summer 1976, (18), 13.

(23) 'Community health programs in the Federated States of Australia', unpublished paper compiled by the Commonwealth Department of Health, Canberra, undated.

(24) Hiddlestone, H. J. H. (Director General of Health, New Zealand, and Chairman of the Executive Board of the WHO), 'Hospital without walls', *World Hospital*, **XVIII** (4), 15–16 Nov 1981; also 'Hospital without walls', *New Zealand Hospital*, **34** (1), 8–9, 12–13 and 16.

(25) Wright-St Clair (Medical Superintendant, Extramural Hospital, Waikato Hospital Board), 'Inside and outside the walls', *New Zealand Health Review*, **3** (1), 7–8, Summer 1983.
(26) Warren, A. D., 'Report on the Extramural Hospital', unpublished paper presented to a group of American health administrators in Auckland, 1981.
(27) *Ibid.*
(28) *Ibid.*
(29) Kaarianinen, H., 'Home care scheme in Helsinki', unpublished (?) paper, Helsinki Municipal Hospital, Helsinki, undated.
(30) Hyde, G., *The Soviet Health Service*, Lawrence and Wishart, London, 1974, pp. 213–5.
(31) Alkalay, L., Letter published in *The Lancet*, 1977, *ii*, 43; Alkalay, L., 'Home Care Unit', in *Kupat Holim Yearbook 1976*, Kupat Holim, Jerusalem, 1976, pp. 95–105.

5 *Hospitalisation à domicile*, France: a first-hand account

Introduction

The French Public Health Code describes the functions of public hospitals thus:

> 'Hospitals provide for the examinations necessary for diagnosis and for preventive medicine, as well as for the treatment (*with or without hospitalisation* [present author's italics]) of the sick, the injured, convalescents, and pregnant women, including . . . necessary functional rehabilitation . . . . They are open to all those whose condition requires their services.'[1]

Hospital amenities in France comprise two main categories of establishment. On the one hand, there are public hospitals which never have a profit-making character. On the other, there are private establishments, themselves divided into two types: those set up and managed by non-profit-making organisations and those which have a profit-making purpose. Conditions of development of these two sectors, public and private, have been defined by a series of so-called 'co-ordination texts'.[2] These have the particular object of subjecting the establishment of any new institution and any extension of an old one to previous approval by the Minister of Health, in order to avoid duplication and thus give greater effectiveness to overall plans for health care.

Amongst all public and private hospitals and clinics in France, it is further necessary to distinguish between general and special hospitals (for example, for fever, mental illness and tuberculosis). The existence of these special hospitals does not, however, prohibit the setting up of corresponding units in general hospitals, provided the need exists.

To set information about the French service of '*hospitalisation à domicile*' (HAD) in context, it is necessary to state several facts about the French system of liberal medicine.[3]

General practitioners work privately (as do most nurses and physiotherapists outside hospital services). They are free to choose their clients, who, in turn, are free to choose them. Such an arrangement clearly has advantages and disadvantages for both sides. Real freedom of choice exists for patients. (From impressions gained by talking to doctors, other health workers and patients, about 15–20 per cent of the population change doctors rather often). GPs do not usually work in group practices, although the number who do so is increasing. Attachment of nurses and health visitors to general practices is not common. Apart from nurses and paramedical workers employed through the liberal sector, many are employed direct by public concerns operating community and domiciliary services.[4]

It is important to understand that 'liberal' medicine in France is in no way equivalent in meaning to 'private' medicine in Britain. The reason is that 'la Securité Sociale', the social security insurance system to which virtually all French citizens are obliged to belong, reimburses all medical and allied expenses approved in an official tariff whether for public or privately run services. This arrangement covers all essential items ranging from consultations, pharmaceutical preparations and nursing and paramedical services to diagnostic procedures, tests, ambulance transport, rehabilitation, the hire of special equipment and the provision of prostheses. The level of reimbursement depends on a number of factors, but in the case of hospitalisation is usually between 80 and 100 per cent. (Patients of the type elligible for admission to HAD are usually reimbursed at 100 per cent.) Since reimbursement rates apply equally to public and private services the private sector is not thought of as being for wealthy patients alone and is, in fact, used by members of all classes and occupations of the French people.[5]

Hospitalisation à domicile[6]

Creation and initial growth

In 1957, an experiment was undertaken by l'Assistance Publique
(the Paris Regional Hospital Authority), to test the possibilities of
providing domiciliary care facilities, parallel in level and variety
to those of its public hospitals, for patients already hospitalised
but not fit for discharge to traditional community care arrangements. The scheme was to apply only to patients expressing a
wish for home as an alternative to hospital care, and then only
when their caring relatives or other members of their own
entourage agreed with the idea. M. R. Tremollière, l'Assistance
Publique's administrator responsible for introducing the idea,
acknowledged the inspiration of Dr Bluestone of Montefiore
Hospital, New York (see pages 57–9).

The experiment entitled 'l'Hôpitalisation (now Hospitalisation) à Domicile' (HAD) began at the Tenon Hospital in the
20th arrondissement (district) of Paris, selected because there
was an acute shortage of hospital beds in the area at the time. It
was designed from the outset to allow for an eventual growth of
separate units within a centralised network to cover the whole of
the Paris region, as and when the demand for it was expressed
locally.

A little later a home care scheme for cancer sufferers was added
to the facilities of the Gustav Roussy anti-cancer institute. This
scheme was introduced independently of the l'Assistance
Publique experiment and has since retained its separate identity.
It has, nevertheless, greatly contributed to the total of home care
facilities in the region.[7] In 1968 a third project called
"l'Hospital à Domicile" was introduced to the private non-
profit-making sector of the Paris hospitals system, providing
similar facilities to l'Assistance Publique's scheme.

Meanwhile elsewhere in France smaller projects, acknowledging directly or indirectly the inspiration of Dr Bluestone, began to
proliferate in localities demographically diverse from those of
Paris and between themselves. By the mid-1970s well over 20
HAD schemes were in successful operation or well advanced in
the planning stages, each reflecting the problems and possibilities
of its own particular area. They included those at Bayonne, Dax

and Pau (in the Basque country), Amiens, Angoulême, Bordeaux, Caen, Dijon, Lens, Lyon, Mulhouse and Nice.

In 1974 the Fédération Nationale des Etablissements d'Hospitalisation à Domicile was set up, reflecting views held in common by all its members as to the concept behind HAD and the organisational arrangements necessary to enable its fulfilment.[8]

In 1970 the pioneering activities of l'Assistance Publique in developing HAD were tacitly acknowledged by the French Government when an Act of great potential significance for the home-bound dependent sick was placed on the statute books. Translated, the Act states: ' . . . hospitals may extend their services to patients in their own homes, to continue treatment with the co-operation of the GP, *provided the patient and the family agree*' [present author's italics]. [9]

Budgetry considerations

Reliance of French hospital services on the fiscal support of the statutory health insurance system of the country obliges hospital authorities responsible for the running of HAD schemes to seek agreement with regional Securité Sociale departments to the introduction of such schemes and, thereafter, to renew, annually, agreements to their continuing operation. The Securité Sociale is interested in three main considerations: whether the schemes provide genuine alternatives to general hospital care through pre-agreed operational procedures; whether they ensure the use of these alternatives by *bona fide* hospital patients only; whether they satisfy these first two considerations within an agreed annual budget, usually of less than half the average cost, per person per day, of the estimated average daily cost of maintaining a general hospital bed in the particular areas. Only if these three conditions are satisfied will the Securité Sociale undertake to make the 80–100 per cent reimbursements for each patient of the current year which finance the schemes for the coming year.

The strict conditions of operation imposed on individual HAD schemes have two important advantages: they oblige schemes to operate with maximum efficiency and regard for their stated aims, thus ensuring patient safeguards; they protect schemes against excessive or inappropriate demands from traditional hospital services wishing to divest themselves of unwanted patients, and from pressures from GPs to accept patients who do not need hospital-level care.

In return for hospital-level reimbursements (made direct to the scheme) HAD schemes are required by the Securité Sociale to provide the following free of charge to the patient: professional services of a nursing, paramedical and social nature; materials, equipment and other supplies (including pharmaceutical) requisite to the patient's care and treatment; transport; x-ray, laboratory and other diagnostic facilities; and *all the essential 'looking after' which cannot be willingly and ably provided by the patient's own entourage.* This last requirement represents a tangible acknowledgement of regional hospital authority powers to provide basic patient support (for example, in housework, cooking, shopping). Most HAD cases qualify for a 100 per cent reimbursement. Where a lower rate applies the patient is often also covered by friendly society or private insurance or qualifies for statutory means-tested assistance.

The exclusion of medical consultation fees from the package (dealt with in the traditional manner through payment by and reimbursement to the patient direct) acknowledges French principles of liberal medicine.

Financial economy of HAD operation compared with that of general hospitals is largely accounted for in three ways: patients liable to require costly installations and high concentrations of medical and nursing skills associated with emergency and high technology procedures are not suitable for admission to the scheme; HAD requires little in the way of capital, maintenance, and administrative expenditure (an estimated 90 per cent of expenditure is on personnel); a major part of the cost of home care is inevitably borne by the family – an important reason why family agreement is essential before admission can take place.

Growth and spread

Wherever HAD schemes in France have been created they have seemingly immediately taken root and flourished; the problem at first being to hold them back until reinforcements are built up, so that their services will not be dangerously diluted through over-demand. Their rapid progress has caused some nervousness amongst the Securité Sociale, regional hospital authorities and doctors, accustomed to more traditional ways of working, who fear that their unfettered development could upset delicate balances of interest. In the effort to avert this, public advertisement by the schemes is not permitted. I have been given to understand by workers in the scheme that knowledge of them is actually suppressed by some doctors and other health professionals, worried that they may supercede traditional services.

Whatever the reasons, despite their popularity, HAD facilities are not yet widely available to the French people. But we recall that, to date, only a relatively small number of hospital authorities have ventured to introduce them; those who have are wary of facilitating patient options to the point where they might upset a well established but nonetheless delicate balance between political and administrative health interests on one side, the liberal medical profession on the other: their financing bodies apply stringent criteria for their use.

I have not had the opportunity to visit in person all HAD schemes in France of which I am aware. My first-hand experience of four, however, is sufficient for me to pass on to readers a fair idea of the way they operate and local regard held for them. My unaccompanied visits date from 1972 onwards, but those of 1977 in joint undertaking with Stephen Cang (see page 54) enabled deeper analysis of the schemes than had hitherto been possible. During that year alone we met in person a total of nearly 150 persons connected with the schemes: their personnel; consultants and GPs using them for their patients; the latter and their families; HAD administrators and insurance officials involved in their regulation and budgetry control.

Our visits included the HAD services of l'Assistance Publique, Paris; l'Hôpital au Foyer, Bordeaux; le Centre Hospitalier Régionale de Grenoble; Santé-Service, Bayonne, in the Basque country.[10]

Scope, levels and varieties of services available under HAD schemes in France are determined according to local conditions. Although their make-up may vary from one to another, their methods of working are remarkably similar, conforming in principle to guidelines agreed by their national federation. These suggest optimal operation through units catering for between 50 and 70 patients at a time. Thus, HAD (Paris) now operates a centralised network of around 25 units, in total providing for about a thousand patients at a time while HAD (Grenoble) provides for around 200 patients through three units and HAD (Bordeaux) rather fewer, through two units.

In principle, prospective HAD patients must first have been hospitalised in units for the acutely ill. An exception has been made in the case of Santé-Service Bayonne. This is because there are few available hospital beds in its area of operation: people of the Basque country are highly resistant to any form of institutionalisation. Santé-Service Bayonne is also different from other HAD schemes in other respects: terrain and demographic features of the area have led to its growth through decentralis-ation, rather than through a tight network as in HAD (Paris); many of its personnel must work in comparative isolation (since travel is difficult, sometimes impossible, in parts of the Basque country, they are as far as possible allocated cases of patients living in their own home areas); dearth of qualified nurses has led to the development of caring teams in which the latter supervise ancillary personnel in a ratio of one to ten (in Paris it is around one to one).

A closer look at HAD (Paris) and Santé-Service Bayonne, with passing reference to the schemes of Grenoble and Bordeaux, gives us a global idea of the possibilities of hospital-based schemes of domiciliary patient care, along the lines of *hospitalisation à domicile*, within the context of nationalised health services.

Hospitalisation à Domicile (HAD), l'Assistance Publique (Paris)

HAD (Paris) headquarters lie in the grounds of Salpetrière Hospital. HQ staff are accountable to l'Assistance Publique for the organisation and operation, within a prescribed annual budget, of a network of HAD units throughout the Paris region.

Each unit is sited in, but not an administrative part of, a district general hospital. Subject to case suitability, patients referred by their hospitals of origin are admitted to HAD units nearest to their own homes. As in London, where teaching hospitals also abound, many patients are admitted to hospitals with high reputations in particular medical specialisms, rather than to their local ones. So a scheme covering a network of 25 hospitals requires potentially infinite numbers of permutations between respective units. To assure both effective administration of the scheme as a whole and day-to-day management of individual HAD cases, units are divided into two sectors: one which deals with admission and discharge procedures and the safeguarding of patients social and financial interests whilst under the scheme; one which assures day-to-day treatment, nursing and basic support of the patient throughout a duration of stay under the scheme. Since HAD is committed to prime consideration of social and psychosocial interests of the sick, in addition to those of a clinical nature, a medical social worker (whose training in France includes important elements of medical and basic nursing knowledge) heads the former. The latter is headed by a nursing officer, whose role extends beyond that of traditional nursing to include management responsibility for the basic (including domestic and social) support of patients placed under her care.

Although separately managed, the two sectors work closely together on mutual cases. When professional nursing advice is required over a matter of admission or discharge, the medical social worker of the HAD referring unit consults with the nursing officer of the receiving unit. When the latter requires professional social worker help over a case she calls upon the responsible medical social worker. But, since the case has already been investigated by the latter at the time of admission, the patient does not rely uniquely on nursing assessment to determine social need.

It will thus be seen that the presence of a central administration, outside traditional hospital in-patient services, is crucial to the concept of HAD, however small the number of units in a particular scheme. It is also crucial to effective and economic practice, ensuring, for example, the economic use of often costly equipment; its maintenance, early repair and replacement when obsolete; appropriate selection, training and induction of personnel; their optimum formation; minimum requisite levels and varieties of services; specialist provision; rationalisation of transport.

When a particular unit has grown too large to react with sensitivity to human needs (both of patients and personnel) it is divided to provide the embryo for another. HAD development in this respect has been particularly impressive in Paris. But in principle it applies equally elsewhere in France.

Admission procedure

An application for an HAD admission might first be prompted by various different bodies. In 1978, a questionnaire circulated amongst 515 patients variously in eight HAD units in Paris found that 10 per cent had become interested in the scheme from what they had learned in their hospital wards, 13.40 per cent through the HAD unit itself, 16.31 per cent from their GPs, 13 per cent from the home and family circle, 4.27 per cent from press reports, 1.96 per cent from community nurses and 2.74 per cent from other sources such as ambulance attendants.[11] Whatever the origin of interest, no referral can proceed without formal application from the doctor presently in charge of the patient's case. If this doctor considers that home care under HAD is medically feasible and is willing to make the formal application, a number of duties must be undertaken by the social worker before an admission can be effected. First, she must make sure that the patient concerned really does want to be looked after at home. (Such a precaution is necessary because it is not unknown for ward doctors and nurses to refer cases to HAD in the hope of moving patients unwanted by themselves, rather than those who have requested the HAD alternative to hospital care.)

The next step is to make sure that the home is suitable and that members of the patient's entourage involved are capable of participating in and in agreement with arrangements proposed. In principle, the presence of a relative or friend living in is required, but in practice, for humanitarian reasons, HAD cares for many patients who live on their own.

Following discussion with the hospital doctor, the patient and caring relatives, the patient's GP must be put in the picture and asked whether he or she would be willing to undertake clinical responsibility for the case according to HAD conditions. If so the social worker refers the case to the HAD unit near the patient's home. From then on HAD social worker (referring unit), nursing officer (receiving unit), GP and ward staff liaise to make practical arrangements for the patient's transfer from ward to sick room at home. The nursing officer discusses case management with ward sister and doctor, and confirms with the social worker arrangements for the supply of materials of a non-nursing nature which may be lacking in the home. They also discuss arrangements and potential problems of a social nature, such as the amount of family support available, prospects of neighbourly help and potential financial and domestic difficulties. (The nursing officer may at this point wish to visit the home herself before committing herself to home care arrangements.) The nursing officer then takes the patient's hospital notes to the GP for up to 48 hours, so that between them they can make up a HAD dossier and the GP can extract information of medical importance. (Here the GP may wish to visit the patient in hospital and confer with the consultant.)

Meanwhile, the social worker confirms Securité Sociale acceptance of financial responsibility for the case, arranges supplies of non-nursing materials and other forms of non-nursing support required, which may have to be negotiated with organisations outside HAD. The patient does not leave the security of a hospital bed until nursing officer and social worker are satisfied that the patient will be similarly protected at home. The whole process is usually completed well within 48 hours of initial referral of a case.

Case management responsibility passes from ward sister to HAD nursing officer at the point where the patient leaves hospital. (If problems are anticipated on the homeward journey an HAD nurse might accompany the patient.) The role of the latter is similar to that of a ward sister, but includes elements which are not present when patients are hospitalised and excludes others which are. HAD nursing involves a delicate balance between professional considerations and patient and family interests which may sometimes apparently conflict with those of a professional nature. Conflict is minimised through precise definition of HAD responsibility vis-à-vis that of the family; definition which is made clear in each case both to HAD personnel and to the patient's entourage. Between these two sides a 24 hour regime is drawn up which assures clinical treatment needs and other elements which are the responsibility of HAD, but which does not interfere more than is inevitable with normal family routines and interests.

Scope, level and varieties of services under HAD depend partly on budgetry considerations, partly on local availability of skills, personnel and resources. Thus the make-up of HAD units may vary greatly from one to another. This does not, however, affect the essential *nature* of HAD, since patients opt for its services in preference to in-hospital care, knowing the limitations of provision likely to apply in their particular cases. It does, of course, affect numbers and types of cases which a particular scheme is able to accept at a given time.

Duration of stay

A doctor making application for a patient stay in HAD must state its estimated duration. This helps nursing officer and social worker determine whether care under HAD is feasible in terms of HAD and family resources available for that period. If, towards its end, the patient is not thought likely to be fit for discharge to traditional community care arrangements, the doctor may make application for an extension, which requires Securité Sociale approval. Estimated duration may vary from only a week or so, where rapid recovery is anticipated, to several months (extendable, even, to years) where recovery is likely to be slow or where no recovery is envisaged. In the latter cases it is a condition of continuous HAD intervention that the patient must be considered by the doctor(s) involved to require continuing regular medical treatment and/or supervision.

Patient and caring aide

On the day of the patient's transfer from hospital ward to sickroom at home under HAD, the nurse allocated charge of the case will either travel home with the patient or await his/her arrival there. The room will by now be comfortably furnished, warm, and equipped to meet the patient's treatment needs. Meals arrangements suited to dietary requirements will have been made. The various carers (family, friends, neighbours and HAD personnel) to be involved in the case will each be aware of their own commitments in relation to those of their colleagues.

Many HAD patients do not have adequate support from members of their own entourages to provide for their 24 hour attendance. This may be unnecessary, unwanted by the patient or impossible in the light of HAD personnel available (perhaps all three). But, if a patient is to be left alone for considerable periods of time, confirmation is sought from the doctor in charge of the case that this is medically permissible. (If not the patient must be hospitalised.)

All caring personnel and the patient (where physically and mentally able to exercise discretion) are fully instructed in steps to take in the event of emergencies. In practice the latter are few and far between because they have usually been anticipated.

A fundamentally nursing-oriented domiciliary service cannot match hospital provision for the sick because it is not equipped or suited to provide elements of basic support outside nursing. At the same time, a domiciliary treatment service expressly for use in cases of major patient dependency must be managed by professionals working to medical prescription: that is, by nurses or paramedical workers. HAD has resolved the problem of providing guarantees of at least minimum adequate basic patient support by extending the role of nursing management to cover personnel whose duties include many traditionally outside nursing (for example, housework, shopping, cashing pensions, changing library books, and otherwise helping the patient to keep warm, comfortable, well fed, psychologically and emotionally fulfilled, and stimulated by outside interests as far as his/her physical condition will allow). These personnel are known as '*aides-soignantes*' – caring aides. All known HAD schemes employ such aides. But the extent of the work they do depends, on the one hand, on the ratio of aides to nurses in a particular scheme; on the other, on the amount of willing and able family support available in a particular patient case.

The *aide-soignante* allocated to a case will be introduced to patient and family and given details relevant to her own work before she is left alone in attendance. Between them nurse, caring aide and family will arrange a daily routine, whereby the aide attends at fixed times for fixed periods. Maximum average daily hours feasible depend on budgetry considerations and personnel available in individual schemes. In Paris, when I visited in 1972, this maximum average was five hours, but this has since had to be reduced in the light of global hospital budgetry cuts in the area and improved working conditions for nurses and ancillary personnel throughout France.) Within the maximum average, flexibility is both highly feasible and desirable. Hours can be amalgamated to provide, for example, a day's respite for a relative, rather than help on a regular daily basis.

Aides-soignantes are selected for personal qualities in caring for the sick, demonstrated perhaps in their previous work as hospital orderlies or in nursing sick members of their own families. Alternatively they may have earlier embarked on nursing or paramedical careers, but failed to qualify, lacking aptitudes of an academic kind, or having left to bring up families. Whatever their backgrounds, these aides must undergo training suited to their individual needs through in-training on a short full-time course and then sessions which take place alongside their day-to-day work, extending over a two-year period. This leads to a certificate of aptitude according them statutory recognition.

The roles of *aides-soignantes* include wide varieties of duties which can perhaps best be described as any which might be carried out by a competent and caring member of the patient's family, were such a person available. The nurse calls daily to check the patient's progress, ensure that relationships between family and aide are going smoothly and to perform nursing procedures of a skilled nature. In the latter she may be assisted by the aide. In the case of need for their intervention, other professionals (for example, social or paramedical workers) might allocate to the aide (with the agreement of the nurse in charge of the case) duties which they feel can be entrusted to her under their own professional supervision.

The role of the doctor

As had been anticipated, the most sensitive aspect of HAD

operation in France has been medical cover for patients, who, by removal from hospital to home, could become remote from their consultants and other hospital doctors acquainted with their cases. Hospital doctors may be doubtful about the ability or willingness of some family doctors to meet clinical responsibilities which they themselves consider necessary. On their sides, family doctors may resent the continued participation of consultants in the conduct of cases for which *they* now hold front-line clinical responsibility. In either case the factor may determine willingness of doctors to use the scheme. At no time during my visits to HAD did I find evidence of problems in following mutually agreed treatment programmes from either side. But then, I met only doctors enthusiastic about the concepts of HAD.

Continuing involvement of the hospital consultant in the case is crucial to the scheme: it is a requirement of the Securité Sociale that the hospital identity of the case be retained; it ensures access to hospital-held resources and skills; it provides for immediate specialist intervention where necessary and reinforces the hospital's commitment to re-admit the patient, as a priority, if the need arises.

HAD ensures continuing GP and consultant participation from both sides: the GP must visit the patient regularly, usually twice a week, in addition to when emergencies arise; the consultant must see the patient regularly, either at home or at the hospital, usually once a fortnight. Traditionally, doctors dislike having to conform with regulations, on the grounds that their patients' medical interests are better assured through their own senses of professional commitment. But since HAD holds overall responsibility for patients admitted to its care, cases where doctors are not prepared to make firm clinical commitments of the above kind cannot be undertaken by the scheme. This is a source of disaffection with the scheme from some doctors, who would like to use it without the conditions attached. They fear the implications of a scheme which might encourage patients whose doctors are *not* prepared to accept the conditions of HAD to go to others who *are* prepared to accept them. The doctors whom I met, however, appreciated the way in which the scheme reinforced collaborative effort between consultant and family doctor, enriching professional experience in addition to enhancing treatment prospects for patients.

Hospital re-admission

Although GPs hold clinical responsibility for their patients in HAD, patient, family, HAD nurse or social worker can request a patient's return to hospital if either party is not satisfied with home care arrangements. If the doctor(s) involved refuse this, HAD may feel obliged in its own interests to withdraw from the case, but such a move is not lightly made. All sides usually get together in an effort to sort out problems which have arisen and try as far as possible to meet the patient's wishes. On a number of occasions when visiting patients with HAD nurses the latter have remarked to me: 'she [or he] really *ought* to be in hospital, but we haven't the heart to make her [or him] go'. Undoubtedly, this can present problems for families, or neighbours where involved, who have to bear the brunt of increasing demands on their resources and time, when those of HAD are already over-stretched. This is an inevitable consequence of enabling more patient participation in decision making than exists under traditional hospital arrangements.

Medical case-notes

The HAD dossier, made up by the scheme's nursing officer at the point of the patient's admission to the scheme, contains records of a medical, nursing, paramedical and social nature and is part of a continuing hospital case-record. Throughout the patient's stay under the scheme, part of the dossier is kept at the patient's bedside and the other part at the unit HQ. On the patient's discharge the notes are amalgamated, to be filed in the regional hospital records so as to be readily available for any future hospital episode wherever this might occur.

Medical arbitration

All HAD schemes have medical consultancy facilities whereby hospital and family doctors can discuss points at issue over the operation of HAD with members of their own profession. In practice, however, contention over case management seldom occurs. HAD staff work harmoniously with the doctors involved in each particular case for which the latter are clinically responsible. Since the Securité Sociate can terminate a HAD arrangement (if, for example, a patient has been cared for under the scheme longer than is customary in his or her type of case), a medical consultant of the Securité Sociale is available for arbitration purposes.

Children

In the latter half of the 1970s a children's unit was introduced to HAD of l'Assistance Publique, Paris. I visited this in 1980, by which time it had established for itself an important place in the continuing care of children suffering major illness. Its six paediatric-trained nurses are sectorised and work under the supervision of a paediatric-trained nursing officer. I did not accompany these nurses on their rounds, as I had in the case of the general units, as the presence of an observer might have been disturbing to the children involved. But, sitting in on one of their daily 'report-ins', I was impressed by teamwork spirit and the way in which needs of families as a whole were considered.

Hospitalisation à Domicile, Grenoble[12]

HAD (Grenoble) differs from HAD (Paris): partly for reasons of size, division into three units is adequate; partly because it is situated in the only district hospital of the area. As a result, its administration, although separate from, has closer collaborative links with other district hospital services than have hospital-based units of HAD (Paris) operating under central administration. Furthermore, the appointment of a medical consultant from the district hospital as its director apparently leads to the forging of closer links with other clinical units of the hospital than is the case in HAD (Paris).

In addition to its three general operational units, HAD (Grenoble) possesses a well established, highly valued, specialist facility for young children and premature babies; there is also a skin unit with specialist staff. It employs a psychiatrist, who, in addition to intervention in individual patient cases where requested by the case doctor, provides support to HAD personnel and advice in case management, through lectures, participation in training programmes and case discussions.

L'Hôpital au Foyer, Bagatelle Foundation, Bordeaux[13]

L'Hôpital au Foyer is the HAD unit of the Bagatelle Foundation, a non-profit-making hospital complex of Protestant origin in Bordeaux. The complex includes a general hospital of 285 beds, a health and social centre, a training school (established through close links with Florence Nightingale), and l'Hôpital au Foyer. Its facilities are open to all patient groups.

The health and social centre has changed significantly in recent years. It still retains its original functions as an out-patient dispensary, but these have now been extended to provide a centre for meetings, seminars and the exchange of ideas. It has provided home nursing services since 1921, but responsibility for these has now been assumed by the public authorities.

The HAD unit – l'Hôpital au Foyer – was created in 1975 in response to an urgent need to provide more comprehensive home care alternatives to hospitalisation than were possible by using the community nurses of the health and social centre, already responsible for a wide range of primary care services.

Apart from providing a service for patients hospitalised in 'Bagatelle' itself, l'Hôpital au Foyer provides for patients of other hospitals of the area. These hospitals must first have reached independent agreement with the local Securité Sociale office to their participation in the scheme.

Santé-Service, Bayonne[14]

Santé-Service Bayonne is of particular interest to British students of 'hospital at home', because it reflects the ability of HAD to modify its provisions to meet demographic needs and possibilities in particular areas.

I first visited the Bayonne scheme in 1974, when, after two years of operation under almost overwhelming difficulties, it had grown so rapidly in the following three years that the problem now was how to hold it back while additional staff were enlisted and trained to provide for its surge of case referrals.

Bayonne lies on the coast of the northern area of the Basque country. In 1974 its general hospital had only 200 beds, a totally inadequate number to meet the treatment needs of a scattered population of 100 000 persons. Outside towns, the Basque people are highly resistant to leaving their homes, where their livelihoods – with meagre crops to be attended to, chickens fed and goats milked – depend on their presence all the year round. Consequently they frequently ignore the need for medical attention, which in any case is difficult to come by.

In the mid-1960s, Dr Thielley, a cancer specialist in Bayonne, resolved to introduce a home care scheme based on the ideas of Dr Bluestone in New York (see pages 57–9) but adapted to the particular needs of the Basque country. At the time he was unaware of the Paris experiment, now providing for almost a thousand patients. (He told me he heard of it by chance when his own plans were nearing completion.)

At first no statutory financial backing was available for the Bayonne experiment: money had to be raised from well-wishers and sympathetic charities. Foremost of these was the French anti-cancer league – le League Nationale Française Contre le Cancer – of which Dr Thielley was the local president.

Santé-Service Bayonne was launched in 1968. During its first two years of operation under charitable funding it managed to satisfy the Securité Sociale as to its capacity to provide a genuine alternative to hospital admission and reached formal agreement to its continuing operation on terms similar to those of other HAD schemes, but with two important exceptions. These concerned conditions of patient eligibility and the basis of financial reimbursement from the Securité Sociale to Santé-Service for patients admitted to the scheme. First, since hospital beds in the area were totally inadequate to allow for hospitalisation prior to admission (and, in any case, patients would have been unlikely to agree to such a condition), it was accepted that they could be admitted direct from their homes. Second, gaining from the experience of a financially disastrous start (caused mainly because Securité Sociale would not accept Santé-Service's original recommendations for the categorisation of patients), it was agreed that the cost of care should be kept to a level similar to that achieved by other HAD schemes through the application of three categories: category 'A' patients could have from 16 to 24 hours attention a day for up to 10 days before review; category 'B' patients could have approximately 12 hours attention per day for an initial period of up to a month; Category 'C', from 2 to 4 hours daily for an initial three months. Category 'A' would cover major medical and paramedical treatment, equipment and materials; 'B', high levels of professional attention and material provision, but less constant attention; 'C', minor medical and treatment needs, little in the way of material provision, and more limited hours of attendance from non-professional staff than in the cases of the other categories. Patients could be transferred from one category to another as the need arose. By regulating numbers of patients admitted to respective categories, annual budgetry balance could be maintained, similar to that achieved by HAD schemes elsewhere accepting only pre-hospitalised patients and with fixed ceilings of staff attendance applicable to all cases. Although it might be less than ideal that some Santé-Service patients should have to be admitted or transferred to categories lower than those they had been assessed to qualify for, they nevertheless gained benefits impossible outside the scheme.

During its first year of operation Santé-Service Bayonne averaged only 17 patients. Five years later it averaged 300, a figure it was finding difficult to hold in check. Lack of funds and available qualified nurses, in a difficult terrain, poorly served for transport, obliged the scheme to seek novel ways of conserving and making maximum use of nursing skills in short supply. This was achieved through the enlistment of *aides-soignantes* (caring aides) in a ratio to nurses of 10 : 1, as against the Paris level of approximately 1 : 1 (see page 76).

It might have been expected that this high ratio of unqualified to qualified staff would dilute the professional element of the service to a point where it was incapable of fulfilling its hospital-parallel identity. But apparently this was not the case. In many respects Dr Thielley found that *aides-soignantes*, carefully selected for their proven caring qualities, trained in minimum essential skills and well supervised, usually living in close proximity to the cases allocated to them, were often more effective in their work than nurses who might resent having to undertake what they regarded as non-nursing duties in their daily rounds.

Like other HAD services, Santé-Service Bayonne has found operation through small personalised units highly satisfying for both patients and staff. When I first visited the scheme in 1974 it was already finding its three units, each of nearly a hundred patients, too large. Plans were afoot for the creation of similar schemes in three other regions of the Basque country. These are now fully operational.

Summary and conclusions

Readers may feel that study of home care experiment under a health system radically different from that of the NHS is of little value to a country already providing community care on a level which has earned world-wide admiration. However, arguably many developed countries, including France, now provide health care equal to, or in advance of, that of the UK, although administrations appear to be more cumbersome, facilities less accessible, in countries without nationalised services. Regardless, of ways in which various overseas health systems are organised, most are seemingly, like the NHS, deficient in their domiciliary provisions for the dependent sick.

From the French experience of HAD we are able to study the application of sound structure and organisation in an attempt to provide genuine domiciliary parallels to general hospital admission – a prerequisite to realistic patient options in environments of treatment. We in the UK continue to rely on piecemeal, *ad hoc* arrangements, even for patients suffering terminal illness.

Following 1974 reorganisation, the NHS lost its capacity for experiment involving structural integration of hospital and community medical and nursing services with personal social services for the disabled sick. Research analysis of HAD (Paris) in

1974, concluded such integration to be crucial to the success of the scheme for both humane reasons and those of hospital bed and cost economy.[15] It also found that level and quality of medical social worker involvement in the scheme directly influences the capacity of HAD nurses to make economic and effective use of skills and resources under nursing control.

It happens like this. As with hospital beds, fresh patients cannot be admitted to HAD until places have been vacated by existing patients. If social workers are too busy making enquiries about new cases to make arrangements for the discharge of existing ones, the latter block places which would otherwise be available for the former. If they concentrate on making arrangements for the discharge of existing patients, they are unable to process new applications. This results in delays in admission which cause doctors, already uneasy about a scheme still in its infancy, and which they may never before have used themselves, to resort to traditional hospital admissions for their patients interested in HAD. In acute cases, delay of over a day or so would have this effect. Discouragement of medical applications for short term admissions defeats the fundamental aims of HAD to provide parallel alternatives to hospitalisation for potentially *all* patients opting for them and whose cases meet medical criteria for admission. (NB: These criteria recognise that no patient can be admitted without the agreement of the doctor who will be clinically responsible for the case.)

Exclusion of acutely ill patients from HAD would lead to concepts of a facility suited only to the needs of long term patients – the elderly infirm and chronically sick. HAD recognises that the needs of such groups must be covered, but distinguishes between their members needing close regular medical attendance and those who, given satisfactory *non-treatment* health and social services could be adequately protected from additionally disabling illnesses through traditional family doctoring. It identifies as its own responsibility the former, because a combination of major chronic disablement and acute illness, however relatively mild, implies need for a service which includes elements of medical treatment, nursing, social and basic support, which can be harnessed in level and variety according to individual patient needs.

HAD has developed a formula for operation which has proved

effective in identifying patients qualifying for its services without resort to often meaningless distinctions between 'geriatric', 'chronic' and 'acute' cases. It is not necessarily the variety of illness or age of patient which determines the kind of service required (it might be a case of influenza or a terminal condition in a person young or old), but rather the effect of illness, taking into account physical, mental and social considerations, through-out its duration. This formula rests on principles of case management which cannot be properly applied if initial assess-ments are made only by doctor and nurse responsible for the patient's daily care because they bear no statutory responsibility for meeting non-medical and non-nursing requirements. Hence the need for a separate social sector, responsible for identifying and meeting essential requirements of other kinds.

When, in 1970, French hospital law reform authorised the extension of hospital services to the homes of patients (see page 73), these authorities were able to make explicit requirements of social workers responsible for the management of HAD assess-ment and social sectors. In addition to specific duties connected with case assessment and formalities of case admission, these social workers provide on-going patient and family support where necessary during a patient stay in HAD and arrange for continuing community support where necessary on discharge. Thus, their presence is crucial to the efficient and economic operation of HAD as well as to the humane interests of its patients.

HAD nurses are emphatic that they could not operate effectively without the presence of social sectors whose social workers are immediately on hand to free them from duties outside their day-to-day nursing and managerial commitments.

The prime value of study of French HAD experiment to the British health worker lies in its demonstration of the need for structure and organisation capable of providing for all essential elements of patient treatment, nursing care and social and domestic support. France has found a formula for domiciliary care which could provide for all patients not obliged to enter hospital for treatment reasons. The extent to which it can be realised depends on willingness of the medical profession to utilise it, and budgetry and staffing feasibility. The more widespread and even its distribution and the greater the number of patients able to opt for it, the greater should be its economy of use per patient-day.

Future HAD growth and development will be determined by a number of factors: its major economy over hospital admission must be demonstrated in its annual budgets; there must be sufficient qualified personnel in a given area to provide both adequate case skills and competent professional management of non-professional workers, who must be available in sufficient numbers to provide high levels of sickroom attendance; doctors must be motivated towards use of HAD facilities for hospital patients opting for them; wide public understanding of HAD concepts and knowledge of its facilities available is required before public pressure is likely to persuade hospital authorities to redress existing imbalance between hospital and domiciliary patient services.

Additionally, there are a number of reasons why patients who could be well cared for under HAD may nevertheless prefer in-hospital treatment: it may give them a sense of security they would lack at home; however high the level and wide the variety of services guaranteed by HAD, the main burden of home care responsibility (at least morally) rests with families of the sick (a responsibility which many are unable and/or unwilling to undertake when hospital admission is available); some patients may not feel confident in their family doctors' capacities to provide the kinds of services envisaged of them by HAD.

Finally, in France, as in other Western and Western-style democracies, medicine is traditionally orientated in favour of hospitals and patient services are organised accordingly. Interests of both medical and nursing professions depend to a large extent on high level maintenance of institutional services viz à viz those of home care. Despite the fact that France has found a formula able to offer parallel domiciliary alternatives to hospitalised patients, questions remain as to how far liberal medical and nursing professionals are prepared for it to be developed.

British interest in French HAD experiment (dating from publication of my first findings in the early 1970s) has been demonstrated by the appreciation of health administrators, academics, doctors, nurses and paramedical workers of a service fundamentally different from any yet provided in the UK. This has also been apparent to members of many community health councils and special patient-interest groups, as well as to others closely affected by illness in the home, or with loved ones hospitalised against their wills and for no good medical reason, because statutory help of the right kind at home has been unavailable.

This interest has given rise to numerous British experiments intended to emulate the French experience. For the most part these have been motivated by hospital bed shortages rather than prime consideration for the wishes of patients themselves. But some organisations, for example, hospices for the terminally ill, have introduced home care facilities to enable continuity of care between hospital and home according to the aspirations of individual patients and their families.

These experiments demonstrate the pressing need in Britain for services similar to those of HAD in France. They also highlight the inability of the NHS in its present form to offer a structure and organisation capable of providing such services.

References and notes

(1) *The French Hospital Service*, French Embassy, London, undated.
(2) *Ibid.*, p. 3.
(3) Cayla, J. S., 'L'exercise liberal de la medicine et l'assurance maladie', unpublished paper, Ecôle Nationale de la Santé Publique, Rennes, 1972.
(4) Cang, S., and Clarke, F., 'Home care of the sick – an emerging general analysis based on schemes in France', *Community Health*, 1978, **9** (3), 167–71.
(5) *Ibid.*
(6) Bibliography on HAD maintained by the Fédération Nationale des Etablissements d'Hospitalisation à Domicile, Paris; information booklet, Fédération Nationale des Etablissements d'Hospitalisation à Domicile, Paris, undated; Clarke, F., 'Hospital at home', *Health and Social Services Journal*, 1973, **LXXXIII** (4338), 1311–2; Chabrin, C., 'L'hospitalisation à domicile', *Médicine et Monde Modèrne*, 15 September 1973.

(7) *Une Realité dans l'Hospitalisation à Domicile*, Santé-Service, Puteaux, Paris.

(8) Information booklet, FNEHAD, *op. cit.*

(9) *Ibid.*

(10) First-hand accounts of these schemes are supplemented by annual reports, statistics, etc., in the present author's possession. Such items include the following: Flores, J., and DeNaurois, J., *Etude sur l'Hospitalisation à Domicile et son Development (l'Assistance Publique de Paris)*, Ecôle Nationale Supèrieure des Mines, Paris, 1975; Duvauchelle, F., 'Hospitalisation à domicile a propos de l'étude du Service d'Hospitalisation à Domicile de Bordeaux', Doctoral thesis, University of Bordeaux, 1977; Thielly, M., 'L'hospitalisation à domicile 'en province' selon l'experience de Santé-Service Bayonne', unpublished paper, Santé-Service Bayonne, Bayonne, 1974 (English translation available from the present author); annual reports for 1971, 1973 and 1977, Hospitalisation à Domicile, Grenoble; *Guide de l'Hospitalisation à Domicile*, Fédération Nationale des Etablissements d'Hospitalisation à Domicile, Paris, undated.

(11) Questionnaire issued by the Fédération Nationale des Etablissements d'Hospitalisation à Domicile, Paris, 1978.

(12) Annual reports of Hospitalisation à Domicile, Grenoble, *op. cit.*

(13) Duvauchelle, *op. cit.*

(14) Thielly, *op. cit.*

(15) Flores and DeNaurois, *op. cit.*, pp. 5, 19–34.

6 Home care experiments in Britain

Introduction

We now return from France to Britain where, by the mid-1970s, economic recession had already begun to take its toll of health and social services, causing public outcry when cuts directly affected hospital provision, but far less overt concern when they led to a lowering of standards of home care for the sick. However, hospital cuts obliged health authorities to turn their attentions to their community sectors, if only to seek cheaper alternatives to unnecessary hospital admissions.

Problems of admission and discharge had taxed health authorities ever since the creation of the NHS, when state welfare provisions and the abolition of the Poor Law largely overcame public resistance to entering hospitals. From then on, a gradual build-up of long-stay patients, usually elderly, led to redesignation of hospital beds and the creation of consultancy posts and units (notably geriatric) designed to free acute beds for acute short-stay cases. The geriatric (and, later, psychogeriatric) medical speciality developed in size and crystallised in concept to the point where, by the mid-1970s, geriatricians up and down the country were able to classify their own unit beds as 'acute' or 'chronic' (short or long stay). They had also established policies and organised their departments in favour of day hospital and out-patient attendance where in-patient care could be avoided. Of all general hospital specialists they had learned the importance of a medico-social approach and the value of drawing into their operation community nursing and personal social services.

In many respects growing emphasis over the past two decades on the establishment of treatment services uniquely for the elderly may have hampered rather than encouraged medical interest as a whole in a medico-social approach to illness. By referring elderly 'problem cases' to geriatricians, other hospital doctors and GPs could persuade themselves they had done their best for patients without taking further action. Moreover, elderly patients themselves often bitterly resent their classification by age, rightly claiming entitlement to treatment on the same basis as patients of any other age groups. Their point is taken when we recall that many 80-year-olds are as spry as others in their 50s. In medical terms we have only to consider how heart disease in the latter can be as calamatous as in those of advanced old age. Additionally, emphasis on special treatment services for the elderly leads to neglect of provision of support facilities more frequently associated with the needs of older people than for patients of younger age groups.

Whether or not such facilities are always *available* for hospital patients, at least their adequate multi-disciplinary treatment and care is *organisationally provided for*. But at home patients must rely on their GPs to mobilise piecemeal *ad hoc* services which may or may not be readily available in their localities. Furthermore, there is no formal requirement of GPs to concern themselves with other than their patients' clinical needs, while hospital out-patient departments provide only for treatments on the spot, or consultations whereby specialists may *suggest* case management and treatment to patients' GPs, but not themselves *prescribe* for them.

Possibilities of providing unified health and social services support for the home-bound patient faded when, in 1973, the NHS Reorganisation Act transferred from health authorities to newly formed local authority social services departments (LASSDs) responsibility for (amongst other stated categories of disadvantaged persons) the social support of the sick. Arguably, this move was of no great significance for hospitalised patients, whose comprehensive needs are automatically covered as a consequence of admission. However, it lent organisational strength to a denial of concepts of unified, comprehensive care upon which the NHS was originally built, but which, in any case, it had never actually put into practice outside its hospital services.

As geriatricians became increasingly selective in the referrals they would accept from their specialist colleagues in the acute medical and surgical units, responsibility was thrown back on the latter to resolve problems of bed-blockage they had originally thought would be resolved through the growth of geriatric units. As a consequence, hospital doctors as a whole began to take more interest in community patient care than hitherto. Their voices were added to those of GPs and community nurses, overtaxed by the problems of patients whom hospitals could not or would not accept and of patients discharged from hospital who were largely incapable of self-help, in a demand for improved community health provision. Since many, perhaps most, of these patients required basic support rather than skilled nursing, a form of organisation was required covering social as well as health services.

Widespread vocal objection to transfer of responsibility for social services connected with health functions from health to local authorities, enacted by the NHS Reorganisation Act (1973) led the DHSS to consider ways in which the interests of patients liable to suffer as a result of divided care could be safeguarded. Accordingly, following reorganisation, it recommended the setting up in each health area of 'health care planning teams'[1] based on population groups of particular concern – for example, children at risk, the elderly infirm, the physically handicapped, the mentally handicapped, and expectant and nursing mothers.

Although these planning teams provided forums for the exchange of views and ideas between hospital and community health personnel and LASSDs, they were of dubious effectiveness in influencing policy decisions determined largely between management and medical committees. Furthermore, divided accountability between central and local government of the personnel involved meant that there could be no guarantee of joint policies which had been agreed being carried out in practice.

I mention these planning teams not for what they did or did not do but for the fact that they effectively excluded from their considerations the main body of patients accommodated in general hospital acute units, of whom, in any case, the majority were the elderly infirm and/or disabled. Furthermore, their functions overlapped: for example, the elderly infirm, the physically handicapped, and the mentally handicapped are three separate groups, but one person patient might easily belong to all three groups. More seriously, cases of a psychogeriatric nature, for example) might be bandied from one group to another.

Joint planning schemes

In 1976, in response to mounting medical pressure for radical solutions to ever increasingly blocked hospital beds, the government announced a scheme for joint health/social services planning which would make specific sums of money available to health authorities for projects which could over a period be taken into local authority responsibility. The scheme was modified in 1977 to clarify arrangements for using the special allocations. The projects would be designed to enable earlier discharge of traditionally hospitalised patients than would have been feasible without them, or to avert their admission altogether. Clearly, access to these schemes had to be extended to all hospital consultants; but, inevitably, their use would be largely confined to the elderly patient. By and large, doctors were not motivated to seek home care alternatives for patients of the younger age groups. Nor yet for old people suffering diseases of special medical interest.

Projects launched according to government guidelines would initially be financed mainly by health authorities. Within a few years, however, the financial burden would fall mainly on the LASSDs operating them. Tempted by prospects of immediate cash injection, not least because they themselves were beset by problems of the elderly infirm inadequately supported at home and for whom accommodation in residential homes was unavilable, LASSDs up and down the country introduced schemes offering health authorities prospects of discharging patients who otherwise would have remained in hospital.[2]

Joint funding was introduced at a time when interest in the experience of *hospitalisation à domicile* in France was widespread. Consequently many authorities drew up plans embodying some of its concepts and criteria of operation. But, for organisational reasons, they could not apply them in similar fashion to French hospital authorities. By definition, they were non-treatment services. Where the French backed their humane approach to patient and family needs with sound structure and organisation, the British schemes would have to rely solely on individuals appointed to operate them: on the one hand, to ensure their strict budgetry regulation; on the other, to protect the interests of patients who, in their absence, would have remained in protective hospital custody. As social support services not covering medical and nursing elements, primarily regarded as services for the chronically sick and disabled, their operational personnel would be highly vulnerable to demands they were not equipped or organised to meet. Their dependence on GPs and community nursing services for items of help which did not fall within LASSD responsibilities meant that they could not guarantee the patterns of comprehensive care which were their aim.

Despite the drawbacks described above, joint funded health/ social services projects have been judged a great advance on hitherto largely unplanned hospital discharges of potentially long term cases. They have brought together, through liaisive and co-ordinative activities, hospital staffs, community health personnel and social services departments, and have been instrumental in bringing specialists and GPs together informally in the clinical management of, for example, geriatric patients. In cases where the wishes of the patient have been the prime factor in deciding between continuing hospitalisation and discharge home, they have proved of great humane patient benefit. Study of some of these schemes confirms this and leaves us in no doubt as to the value placed on them by their operational staffs.

Despite qualified success, joint funding has brought to LASSDs difficult problems of case classification among their own clientele. When a LASSD-operated scheme enables the discharge of a potentially long term hospital patient, the hospital is released from custodial responsibility for the case – a responsibility it will be unlikely to re-assume unless there are fresh medical symptoms to justify it. Patients' families who feel that they have been manipulated, by the presence of a scheme, to undertake more in the way of patient support than they can readily provide, are reluctant to accept in due course its withdrawal of enhanced support in favour of traditional, low-level, *ad hoc* services, which might fluctuate from day to day. Furthermore, as LASSD services made available through joint funding are provided free of charge (on the grounds that without them the patient would have remained in hospital), imposition of means testing for lower levels of support when these services are withdrawn is certain to cause resentment. At the same time, since judgement about who is and who is not entitled to cost-free services is largely empirical, it sometimes happens that cases (perhaps in the same street) with similar needs are treated in wholly dissimilar ways, a situation bound to foster ill feeling.

The main achievement of jointly funded home care schemes has been their demonstration, where the sick and disabled are concerned, of the illogicality of divided health and personal social services. This has stimulated government and administrative thinking about the differing organisational requirements of, respectively, treatment and non-treatment services. So far this has not been reflected in organisational changes. This would require fundamental changes in relationships between GPs and specialists, hospital and community sectors of the NHS, and centrally governed health services and local government personal social services.

Geriatric continuing care programmes

During the 1970s, geriatric units of many health authorities in the UK became focal points for the operation of multi-disciplinary continuing care hospital/community programmes. These have now become so well established that they provide bases on which enhanced budgetry allocations in favour of geriatric departments are largely determined. This is a marked advance on policies of the past whereby numbers of hospital beds alone were the main indications of growth in favour of geriatric specialisation.

Geriatric involvement in the community care of the elderly has not met with the kind of resistance from GPs which might be accorded to other hospital specialists attempting to introduce policies which, these GPs might claim, encroach upon their own professional territories. This is because GP services are overtaxed by problems of the elderly infirm not of interest to the main body of hospital consultants. Individual GPs therefore welcome initiatives from their local geriatric departments which lighten their own burdens of responsibility. At the same time, these initiatives, often relying on extensions of day hospital provision at costs in numbers of hospital beds, have added to the problems of GPs unable to resort to traditional hospitalisation for many of their aged patients. After all, it is the GP, not the geriatrician, who has to respond to the emergency calls of these patients and to attend to their many needs not met by day hospitals and home visits from the latters' nursing, social and paramedical worker personnel. It is the practice-attached district nurse who has to take the strain of heavy home-nursing requirements and social services staff who bear the brunt of basic support. Above all, it is families of the sick who, by the presence of these initiatives, have often found themselves inescapably compromised by arrangements not of their choosing.

Many geriatric initiatives of the kind described above have been inspired wholly with the aims of relieving hospital beds and/or professional advancement in the geriatric field. But some merit special attention because they have been built on essentially humane motives of enabling elderly patients and their families to exercise optimum choice between home and institutional care. Sadly, their realisation has often fallen far short of hopes and expectations, partly for the obvious reasons of staff and resource shortage, but also for less openly acknowledged problems related to fundamentally faulty NHS organisation which no health authority is in a position to overcome. Resistance, principally from doctors and nurses, to departures from traditional ways of working, has also contributed to disappointingly low development and limited spread of ideas of great potential benefit to the elderly.

One of the best known early pioneers of geriatric initiative in the home care of the sick is Dr Monica Stewart, who in the early 1970s, during her appointment in the Geriatric Unit of Edgware General Hospital, Middlesex, introduced to her earlier pioneering work ideas based on the French experience of *hospitalisation à domicile*. In particular, she hoped to develop, in the direction of home care, the work of 're-ablists' – multi-disciplinary paramedical worker aides who for some years had been effectively engaged in the hospital rehabilitation of geriatric in-patients. In the French experience of *aides-soignantes* she foresaw possibilities whereby many such patients might be more effectively re-habilitated in their own homes, through reinforcement of the basic support provided by families, enhanced by hospital-taught rehabilitative skills.[3]

In 1976, Professor J. Williamson of Edinburgh (and previously Liverpool) University, already widely renowned for his advancement of humane geriatric care, set up a control study on the home management of elderly patients.[6] Following publication of *Going Home* – Age Concern's report on research into continuing care for the elderly conducted by Liverpool University – the Continuing Care Project of the Department of Geriatric Medicine at Queen Elizabeth Hospital, Birmingham, sponsored teams of graduates to investigate problems of patients discharged from hospital and of blocked hospital beds.[7] In 1977 Dorset Area Health Authority put forward proposals for a hospital at home project, based on the needs of mentally ill elderly patients of King's Park Hospital; and in the same year, the Department of Geriatric Medicine of Cambridge Area Health Authority called a conference representative of health and social workers from many parts of the country, on the subject of home care for the elderly sick. Also in 1977 the Northern District of Sheffield Area Health Authority (Teaching) put into practice enterprising plans for organised volunteer help where paid help could not be made available to elderly patients at home.[8] In 1976 the British Association of Service to the Elderly chose 'Hospital at Home' as the theme of its annual conference. In 1978 North Tees Health District, Cleveland, introduced a pilot scheme in favour of home in preference to hospital care for the elderly.

Initiatives described above recognised the importance of respecting the wishes of patients and their families in exercising options between hospital and home care, acknowledging that this should not be uniquely the prerogative of the patient's doctor. That these initiatives did not lead to the setting up of schemes capable of affording patients' realistic choice was frequently held to be due to staff and resource shortages. Many of those involved in attempts to set up such schemes would agree that organisational problems were often as much or more to blame.

Sick children

Hospital-based home care schemes for children have been in existence in Britain for nearly 30 years. St Mary's Hospital, Paddington, appears to have been the first hospital in any country to acknowledge the inspiration of Dr Bluestone in New York (see pages 57–9) when, in 1954, it opened its Home Care Unit for Sick Children. At the time there was a high incidence of infectious disease at the hospital and great pressure on beds. A survey had indicated that 30 per cent of child admissions could have been avoided, had home care facilities, linking hospital staff and resources with those of GPs and health and welfare services, been available.[9]

Although dangers of child infection and shortage of hospital beds undoubtedly eased the introduction of the Paddington scheme, clear exposition of the intention behind it and its mode of operation ensured that it would be used only in circumstances favourable to the child. Initially the unit was staffed by a senior and a junior medical registrar and attached medical students and four nurses, providing a 24 hour service. During its first two years of operation it undertook the care of 582 children living within a 3 mile radius of the hospital. Although there has been little change in the number of cases undertaken since 1961, the scope of the scheme has now been considerably reduced. Since 1961 it has operated on a 'nine to five', five day week basis, with only one registrar, one nurse and a part-time secretary. The original aim was to keep the sick child out of hospital and referrals were almost entirely from GPs. After ten years the emphasis changed. Referrals came mainly from hospital doctors, two-thirds of the cases being of a 'chronic' nature. A major reason for this change of policy was a dramatic fall in the incidence of acute infectious disease, increased resistance resulting from improved social conditions, energetic immunisation programmes and the widespread use of antibiotics.[9]

In 1955 Birmingham Childrens' Hospital introduced a home care scheme similar to that of St Mary's Hospital, Paddington. By the end of the 1960s Southampton General Hospital, the Royal Victoria Infirmary, Newcastle-upon-Tyne, and Rotherham, Yorkshire, had followed suit. During the 1970s other hospitals, including the Royal Hospital for Sick Children, Edinburgh, and the Queen Elizabeth Hospital, Gateshead, introduced home care schemes in their areas. The latter appears to have produced the most integrated scheme. Its provisions range from those of traditional hospital facilities, to assessment and out-patient centres, a toy library run in conjunction with the nursery centres of the town and specially trained district nurses who visit the children at home up to three times a day, but not at night. If the visiting nurse considers it necessary, a hospital admission can be arranged without further reference to a doctor. The scheme has strong links with the local social services department. It is calculated that the Gateshead scheme prevents one out of six potential admissions to hospital in the area.

'Children, particularly very young children, should only be admitted to hospital when medical treatment they require cannot be given in other ways without real disadvantage. This may seem obvious, but it is a consideration which should always be in the minds of those responsible for the admission of children to hospitals and evidence submitted suggests that it is still overlooked' (*The Welfare of Children in Hospital*, HMSO, London, 1959).

Governments have long been aware of the damage to sick children which removal to hospital may incur. Far fewer admissions now take place than was the case a quarter of a century ago; but there has been remarkably little advance in positive action to support parents in the care of their sick children at home. Offical attitudes on the subject are vague:

Wherever it is possible, children should be treated in their own homes under the care of the family doctor with help from the services of the local authority and attention at the hospital out-patient department if necessary. Treatment of the child as a day-patient may be helpful' (*Hospital Facilities for Children*, H. M. (1971) DHSS Circular, section 22 Annex).

Evidence to the Court Committee (1974) from the National

Association for the Welfare of Children in Hospital states the following:

> 'It is our belief that many more children could be nursed at home if their parents were sure of supportive services from general practitioners and the nursing services, either available to the parents on call from the hospital or from the community services. This implies that domiciliary medical care from *both general practitioner and consultant paediatrician should be available at all hours*' [present author's italics]

Where health authorities have extended their paediatric services extramurally, GPs can, if they wish, co-ordinate their work with that of specialists towards more and better home care of the sick child. Arrangements can be made whereby parents worried about a sudden change in a child's condition can call on the paediatric department at any time of the day or night and if they wish have the child admitted immediately without the normal (time-taking) procedures. By and large, however, GPs do not respond sympathetically to parental anxiety in the presence of child illness. Their reliance on night call agency and rota arrangements means that they often do not see their patients at times when their background knowledge of the family is most needed. Concerned that their GPs may not respond promptly and sympathetically to a call for a home visit, many parents present their sick children to hospital casualty departments. Here the doctor on duty may not be sufficiently experienced, or have time, to investigate the case fully and make paediatric referrals where appropriate.

By and large, existing home care schemes for sick children work well where families are comfortably placed and parents are articulate and well versed in their welfare entitlements. Their reliance on liaison and co-ordinative arrangements between hospital and community services rather than on a single responsible organisation, however, makes them vulnerable to fluctuations and uncertainties potentially dangerous to many sick children who, nevertheless, suffer separation from home and family as a result of hospitalisation.

Hospital-based domiciliary provision for the disabled

Most disabled persons are looked after by their families, perhaps helped by community nursing and social services. When necessary they are attended by their GPs or referred to hospital out-patient departments – just like everyone else. They rightly resent being considered permanently 'sick'. But, whereas most illness among the normally active does not vitally affect capacity for self-care, even a mild illness in a disabled person can cause immediate breakdown of life-style already modified to cope with disablement. In the absence of domiciliary treatment services capable of responding quickly and competently to the increased demands of illness, the patient frequently has to be hospitalised, regardless of personal wishes. Sometimes this leads to increased immobility of the patient and to breakdown in established patterns of family life.

There now exist many non-statutory home care schemes for the disabled, designed to supplement community nursing and social services with those of a voluntary kind, with the aim of avoiding unwanted hospitalisation. In some instances specialist hospital services are additionally required. The NHS makes limited domiciliary provision for example, in home renal dialysis. But, by and large, it has been left to individual initiative and supplementary funding from outside the health service to ensure round-the-clock provision for domiciliary patients requiring special care. Resulting schemes are few and far between. But they provide us with sterling examples of the comprehensive, integrated approach necessary in the presence of major illness in the home.

The Responaut Service of the South Western Hospital Respiratory Unit of St Thomas' Hospital in London[10] assumes responsibility for the home care of its patients living within a 30 mile radius of the centre. Only 15 or so patients at a time can be cared for in this way, as the service is highly personalised, requiring the allocation of two full-time aides to each case covering every 24 hours. Responauts are wholly dependent for survival on respiratory machines. Their aides are carefully selected for their caring qualities and are trained to look after both patient and machine, and to take emergency action where necessary. A professional team is always to hand: first, to assess case suitability, investigate family circumstances and ensure that the home is modified to meet the needs of a case; thereafter, to advise, supervise and provide professional assistance, when the need arises.

Terminal illness

The most impressive advances in the care of patients at home in recent years have been in the field of terminal illness. These owe much to the inspiration of Dr Cicely Saunders of St Christopher's Hospice, Sydenham, London.[11] Dr Saunders is a qualified nurse and social worker who took up medicine in order to develop her work in the care of the dying. Her pioneering work in this respect is now so widely acknowledged throughout the world that it is exceptional to read any report of overseas development in terminal care which does not recognise her unique contribution.

St Christopher's Hospice is a 54 bed hospital of religious foundation which has now extended its work to the homes of patients so that they can move freely between hospital and home according to personal inclination, family interests and medical and nursing possibilities. Care is based on team effort, comprising doctors, nurses, social workers, volunteers, religious workers and the patient's family, and extends to the support of the family through bereavement. Members of the family are encouraged to help in the care of the patient in the hospice and hospice staff are available to help and advise the family when the patient is at home.

Of all medical conditions, terminal illness attracts the greatest interest in home care for essentially humane reasons. There is little question of finding alternatives to hospitalisation in order to relieve blocked beds. (Although it is not unknown for some hospitals to press for the discharge of some terminally ill patients who linger for longer than has been anticipated!) During the past decade the work of St Christopher's and other hospices like it has attracted massive interest, including financial, from the National Society for Cancer Relief (NSCR).[12] This has enabled the setting up of continuing care units for the terminally ill in many areas not covered by the provisions of hospices – for example in Oxford, Northampton, Northwood (Middlesex), Southampton, Dundee, Aberdeen, Nottingham, Norwich, Cambridge and Swansea. In addition, such units have been established at existing hospices desirous of extending their activities to the patient's home but lacking the funds to do so – for example at St Joseph's Hospice, Hackney, London, St Columba's, Edinburgh, and St Luke's, Sheffield. In the spring of 1982 the number of such services financed by the NSCR totalled 60.[13]

For many years the NSCR has provided cash grants to patients suffering from cancer on recommendation from a medical social worker. This has been available for 'items' of help: perhaps for additional clothing, convalescent or nursing home fees, extra comforts or heating. It has found in the development of its MacMillan Continuing Care Units (Sir Douglas MacMillan was the founder of the NSCR) the means of adopting a structured approach to the needs of the terminally ill, rather than one which relies largely on the perspicacity of individual social workers to identify need and ensure its satisfaction.

A major part of the work of hospices and other terminal care units lies in the complex problem of pain control. It has proved difficult for specialists in this field to persuade some GPs and hospital doctors that optimum pain control is not always within the competence of general practitioners. The work of continuing care units, together with the appointment of oncologists to general hospital posts, has enhanced prospects of minimal suffering amongst the terminally ill both in hospital and at home. There is, however, growing recognition of problems of pain control which apply also to members of other patient groups – for example, sufferers from rheumatism and arthritis. Some terminal care units have now extended their facilities to members of these other groups. However, they represent only a very small fraction of patients accepted. Conditions like rheumatism and arthritis usually imply long-term care, causing blockage in units relying on rapid bed turnover for their optimum operation.

All continuing care units for the terminally ill acknowledge that they cannot intervene in the home care of their patients unless this meets the approval of the GP in the particular case and the readiness of the district nurse to participate in programmes of shared responsibility. Moreover, they are dependent on the willingness and capacity of local authority services, such as of home help, to provide concentrated basic support, often at very short notice, where this is lacking from within the family.

Night-nursing services

Most health authorities provide night-nursing for patients who are terminally ill. But few go so far as to pre-plan this. It is usually organised at short notice through reference to nursing 'banks', whereby nurses living locally and willing to provide their services on an occasional basis can be approached in turn to see if they might be immediately available to attend a particular case. The facility is usually funded in part by the health authority and in part by the Marie Curie Nursing Foundation. It is often assumed that Marie Curie nurses are specially trained to meet the needs of the dying cancer patient. This is seldom the case. They are unlikely to possess special expertise, unless from experience through working on such cases over many years. Even then, they rely on the GP (who may not be experienced in pain control) for patients' prescription needs. Nevertheless, Marie Curie nurses provide a much-valued service as an extension of primary health care, enabling many dying patients who otherwise would have been hospitalised to remain with their families.

The weight of responsibility under such conditions still rests with the family, sometimes increasing moral pressures on the latter for commitments they are neither mentally nor physically equipped to sustain. Available funds seldom permit the presence of a nurse in the home more than two or three times a week, and then only for a few weeks at the most. Marie Curie nurses do not (officially) perform tasks of a menial nature (for example, the washing of soiled bed-linen) any more than do district nurses.

Local experiment in more structured night care in the home than can be provided from a nursing bank alone is characterised by the example of the Bletchley Night Nursing Pilot Scheme, launched by Buckinghamshire County Council in 1973.[14] The scheme was devised prior to NHS reorganisation and hence embodies some of the comprehensive approaches to domiciliary patient care which now rely on health/social services liaison.

Extended general hospital care

Most health authorities with problems of general hospital bed shortage appear to have developed to some extent their community nursing services with a view to reducing hospital stays of patients who have undergone minor surgery and/or whose medical conditions are not of a complex nature. District nurses enjoy the opportunities which such an arrangement offers them to develop skills they may not have exercised since leaving their hospital posts. The early discharge of patients who need major basic support in addition to items of skilled nursing, however, usually arouses their protest. They are neither organised nor equipped for this and consider it unethical of their hospital colleagues to discharge patients with major basic care needs, even at the requests of the latter.

In 1977 the Service Planning Division of the South East Thames Regional Health Authority saw the situation differently. Inspired largely by Dr Lindsay Elliott, a community physician in the Medway District, it introduced its Extended Hospital Care Scheme in the Medway District. This sought to provide facilities for the basic care, in addition to the skilled nursing, of its patients. Its Interim Report, published in October 1978, describes its successes and some of the problems it encountered.[15] This was the first controlled research experiment introduced under the NHS which recognised in concrete form community nursing responsibility to ensure the basic support of patients at home.

Drawing on the experience of *hospitalisation à domicile* in France, the Medway scheme extended the duties of selected nursing auxiliaries to enable the provision of more comprehensive programmes of care than traditionally apply in community nursing. The roles of nurses responsible for these programmes were extended to include the management of personnel now with 'non-nursing' as well as nursing duties.

The only firm conclusion reached in the Interim Report of the

Medway scheme was its popularity with patients. However, from the limited information gained from a questionnaire circulated to health staff, it won the whole-hearted approval of ward sisters; consultants felt they could make more use of it than they had to date; GPs were favourably impressed; and district nurses felt they had not had enough patients on the scheme to pass judgement.

In contrast to the approach adopted by HAD in France, whereby diagnosis was not taken to be of primary significance, the Medway scheme approached the subject of extended care from a diagnostic angle, concluding that it should be possible to arrive at an optimal hospital/extended hospital care length of stay for the commoner diagnoses. It recommended investigation into ways in which patients put on the waiting list for cold surgery could be simultaneously booked for extended hospital care, thus confirming its diagnostic bias.[16]

Clearly, there are important reasons why the Medway scheme cannot extend its services to patients whose needs for basic support are appreciably more than can normally be provided by the primary care services upon which it relies so heavily. Despite its popularity with those patients whose diagnoses meet its criteria for admission, it does not and cannot provide the structure and organisation necessary for the home care of patients of potentially all medical conditions requiring major basic and social support in addition to items of treatment and nursing.

Community hospitals

Community hospital experiment is not strictly relevant to this book, because 'hospital at home' seeks to provide alternatives to *general* hospital admission whereby specialists are involved in case management. It must, however, be mentioned because there will be occasions when, given a community hospital in their area, patients might prefer it as an alternative to both general hospital *and* 'hospital at home' admission.

Community hospitals are different in concept from the cottage hospitals of pre-NHS days and from outlying units of general hospitals used for 'overspill' reasons. The difference lies in the fact that they are exclusively GP amenities wherein specialist care is not available and specialist consultation is only at the specific request of the GP attending a case. There is a tendency for community hospital beds to be monopolised by GPs having an exceptional interest in following through their patient cases. This means that patients of other GPs in the area do not, by and large, enjoy their facilities.

In 1969 a 15-bed ward at Peppard Hospital, one of the peripheral hospitals in the Reading Group, was opened to provide GPs working from a local health centre with facilities for the in-hospital care of patients for whom they considered general hospital facilities unnecessary. It later extended its services to other GPs with practices in the area. By 1973 it had also opened a day ward adjacent to its pilot ward. In the meantime a new community hospital was built on the existing site of the Wallingford and District Hospital, while plans went ahead for the establishment of similar services in Witney and Corby.[17]

Although they do not themselves include specialist services, community hospitals aim to provide common meeting grounds for consultant and GP, thus helping to bridge the gap between specialist hospital and community. Four factors are seen as essential for success: rehabilitation-minded GPs; a unified nursing service for hospital and community; good physiotherapy services; enthusiastic voluntary services serving both hospital and community.

Community hospitals, like all NHS in-patient services, provide basic support for their patients as part of their custodial responsibility. They do not have to contend with issues of principle in relationships between specialists and GPs – these are matters for individual specialist/GP conscience. They have, however, identified two elements which rely for their most effective operation on organisational arrangements cutting across traditional hospital/community boundaries – those of nursing and voluntary support.

Community hospitals are doubtless of inestimable value in providing alternatives to general hospital admission for patients who prefer them to home care and do not require specialist attention. They cannot, however, meet the needs and aspirations of patients requiring hospital-level care but resistant to hospital admission of any kind.

Voluntary home care schemes

In an effort to bridge gaps in statutory home care provision for the sick and/or disabled, numerous schemes inspired and run by dedicated volunteers have been in vigorous operation over many years. In most areas, organisations with an interest in a particular field of disease (for example, multiple sclerosis, rheumatism and arthritis, ileostomy and colostomy) include home visiting and support in their many activities. But more recently local schemes have been set up with the specific intention of co-ordinating the work of volunteers with that of families, doctors, nurses and social workers towards programmes of total care in the home for patients who do not wish to be institutionalised.

Crossroads, a registered charity originating in Rugby, began by chance in 1971. Noel Crane, a gear specialist at Chrysler's factory, dived into the sea off the North Wales Coast and broke his neck. On his discharge from hospital he was looked after by his mother. He was following the television series *Crossroads*, which at the time featured a young man paralysed after an accident. Feeling that the presentation was not authentic, he contacted the producer of the series, who, when he visited Noel to discuss the matter, noticed the strain on his mother of his unrelieved support.[18]

The encounter led to the financing of a two-year project by the television channel broadcasting the series, the idea being to organise a team of paid helpers who could lift some of the burden from relatives caring for the severely disabled. For several years Mrs Pat Osborne, a Rugby district nurse at the time, acted as unpaid organiser of the scheme. It was so successful that the Department of Health and Social Security (DHSS) was persuaded to back it.

In 1977 the European Economic Community (EEC) approved a grant of £100 000 to enable its extension as a trust, under the directorship of Mrs Osborne, to six selected local authorities in the UK. For each participating local authority the DHSS (or the Scottish or Welsh Offices) agreed to boost local schemes by matching funds put into the project by local social services departments involved.[19] Crossroads stresses that the people it helps are not 'patients' as they are not ill. Not being a treatment service, it is thus radically different in concept from 'hospital at home'.

In other areas GPs have acted as catalysts in the establishment of volunteer services aimed at relieving families of burdens of sickness and disability among their members. In 1974, the late Dr Acheson, followed by Dr A. Allibone, initiated a self-help enterprise in Blakeney, Norfolk, financed by local fund-raising activities and later by a grant from the Nuffield Provincial Hospitals Trust. This led to the setting up of the Glaven District Caring Committee, a practical working group which, by 1977, was helping over 800 frail, elderly people in the neighbour-hood.[20] At around the same time Care Unlimited[21] was set up following the inspiration of Dr J. Baker, a GP in Tonbridge, Kent, aimed more specifically at providing help on a short-term basis to relatives caring for the severely ill, often dying, members of their families. Whereas the Crossroads scheme has been able to pay its helpers, organisations such as the Glaven Caring Committee and Care Unlimited rely on voluntary commitment.

Describing the duties of Care Unlimited's helpers, Dr Baker says, ' . . . their job is to sit with the patient, to move him or her in bed as needed, to supply medicine and drinks as needed, and, in general, to tend. I could as well use the word nurse, but this word has implications with regard to training which prohibits its use.' Stressing the need for better care facilities for the sick and dying at home, Dr Baker adds, 'In no sense am I conducting a campaign against hospices, but rather would wish to work more closely with those that exist. I am against spending money on bricks and mortar, when the beds already exist.'[22]

Problems of discrete home care provision

I have described above the wide range of home-care schemes for the sick in Britain in an attempt to give readers an idea of numbers and varieties of different organisations behind them. They have added immeasurably to the humanising of patient care in ways impossible under traditional health and social services.

Discrete alternative provision for a potentially important percentage of the traditionally hospitalised population is, however, administratively and operationally wasteful of skills, personnel and resources, which might be applied to better patient advantage through centralised organisations operating small, personalised, local units able to call on specialist services according to individual case need.

Britain has a proud reputation for leadership in its primary health care services – a reputation now equalled or surpassed by some other developed countries. Its roots of home attendance on the sick, however, lie mainly in personal dedication and effort, directed at individuals or isolated groups. Present-day community nurses here reflect this spirit but lack the organisational means of providing the kinds of care they know many patients in their localities require. NHS provision for the integration and rationalisation of the many continuing hospital/home care initiatives described above would enable potentially all traditionally hospitalised patients resistant to institutional care to benefit from home care alternatives without loss of access to specialist services.

References and notes

(1) Levitt, R., *The Reorganised Health Service*, Croom Helm, London, 1977, pp. 71, 74, 82–4, 86.

(2) *Ibid.*, pp. 22–5, 31–5, 62–5, 69, 72–4, 78–81, 86–7.

(3) Stewart, M., *My Brother's Keeper?* 2nd edn, Health Horizon Ltd, London, 1968.

(4) Clarke, F., 'Hospital at home', *Health and Social Service Journal*, 1973, **LXXX** (4338), 1311–2.

(5) Follis, P., 'Hospital at home', *Pulse*, 6 December 1975.

(6) Between 1973 and 1976, Professor Williamson conducted two pilot studies on home care for the elderly sick in Liverpool. These studies were followed by further ones when Professor Williamson moved to the Department of Geriatric Medicine, University of Edinburgh.

(7) *Continuing Care Project*, Department of Geriatric Medicine, Queen Elizabeth Hospital, Birmingham, 1978; *Going Home – A Continuing*

Care Project of Age Concern, Age Concern, Liverpool, 1975. Also correspondence with the present author.

(8) *Proposals for a Hospital at Home Service in Sheffield*, report presented to the Northern District of Sheffield Area Health Authority (Teaching), 1977.

(9) In October 1974 the National Association for the Welfare of Children held a conference at which the experience of six home care services was reported (St Mary's Hospital, Paddington; Birmingham Children's Hospital; Southampton Children's Hospital; Royal Victoria Infirmary, Newcastle upon Tyne; Queen Elizabeth Hospital, Gateshead; Rotherham, Yorkshire): evidence was collated and presented to the Court Committee. See also the following references: Hunter, M. H. S., 'Paediatric hospital and home care – integrated programmes', *Nursing Times*, 10 March 1973, 33–6; Jenkins, S. M., 'Home care scheme in Paddington', *Nursing Mirror*, **140** (9), 68–70.

(10) Information provided by the Phipps Respiratory Unit, St Thomas' Hospital, London, 1976.

(11) Stoddard, S., *The Hospice Movement*, Jonathan Cape, London, 1979, see pp. 23, 170, 188, 192 (Dr Cicely Saunders), pp. 10–11, 195 (the hospice concept), pp. 66, 71–6, 91, 94–6 (St Christopher's Hospice).

(12) The progress of the MacMillan Units of the National Society for Cancer Relief is reported regularly in the society's quarterly publication, *Cancer Relief News*.

(13) *Cancer Relief News*, Spring 1982.

(14) Marett, D. L., *et al.*, 'Bletchley Night Nursing Pilot Scheme', unpublished report, Buckinghamshire County Council Nursing Service, Aylesbury, 1973.

(15) Armstrong, D., and Elliott, L. M., 'Balance of care', unpublished paper, South East Thames Regional Health Authority, Service Planning Division, London, 1974; Elliott, L. M., *et al.*, *Interim Report of the Extended Hospital Care Scheme in the Medway Health District*, South East Thames Regional Health Authority, Service Planning Division, London, 1978; Pigache, P., 'Who goes home?' *World Medicine*, 30 November 1977, 93–100.

(16) Armstrong and Elliott, *op. cit.*; Elliott *et al.*, *op. cit.*

(17) Hasler, G. C., *Looking Forward: The Community Hospital Concept*, Royal Society of Health, London, 1973, pp. 184–90; Bennett, A. E., 'Community hospitals and general practice', *Update*, June 1975, 1397–1400.

(18) Weightman, G., 'Care at the crossroads', *New Society*, 18 November 1976, 367–9; Weightman, G., 'Home caring', *New*

Society, 4 August 1977, 233; Hudson-Evans, R., 'Quality of life', *British Medical Journal*, 1976, *ii*, 48.

(19) Weightman, 'Care at the crossroads', *op. cit.*

(20) Alibone, A., 'Community conscience leads to caring', *Age Concern*, Spring 1977, 13; 'Summary of conclusions and proposals of the Glaven District Community Project', unpublished report, Glaven District Community Project, Blakeney, 1974.

(21) Baker, J. W., Letter to the editor of *The Guardian*, 3 March 1978; Baker, J. W., 'Care Unlimited: aims and achievements', unpublished report, Care Unlimited, Tonbridge, 1978.

(22) Baker, 'Care Unlimited: aims and achievements', *op. cit.*

(23) Information on 'Home Care' from the Social Services Department, London Borough of Lewisham; Dexter, N., 'Intensive care at home – a report on the work of the jointly financed Home Care Scheme of Avon County Council and Avon AHA', *Health and Social Services Journal*, 13 February 1981, 170–2; Bath, S., 'Bringing it all back home in Barnet', *Community Care*, 2 October 1981, 16–17; Bamford, T., 'Security is an alarm – a report on Harrow Social Services experimental Home Care Scheme', *Health and Social Services Journal*, 13 March 1981, 297–8; Hunt, S., 'The home that Jack built – report on a home care research project by Coventry Council Social Services Department', *Community Care*, 16 February 1977.

7 Peterborough District Hospital at Home three-year pilot scheme

Introduction

A brief account of overseas home care experiments in chapter 4 and a more detailed account of the French experience in chapter 5 suggests that the provision of home care alternatives to hospital admission is widely regarded overseas as the responsibility of hospital, not community, sectors of respective health systems. Broadly, recent British experiment of a similar kind reflects the NHS concept that, however complex and heavy, patient care in the home must be a community (primary) care responsibility.

There is a widely held belief that British primary care provision is more advanced than that in most other developed countries. Certainly, this is the case compared, for example, with that of the USA; and it might have been so a quarter of a century back in other Western democracies. Now, apparently, standards of primary care are roughly similar throughout most EEC countries, although delivery arrangements vary.

In the UK, reliance on independently contracted GPs for preventive, in addition to treatment, services has inhibited NHS development from incorporating certain advantageous features of some overseas health systems without loss of advantages particular to it. The fact that GPs in Britain cannot participate in general hospital work (except under informal arrangements between individual GPs and specialists) implies loss of medical skills and opportunities in the mainstream of curative medicine, whilst doing nothing to assure the optimum interests of prevention.

Home care experiments in Britain such as described in chapter

6 have not been able to parallel the cohesive structures of French *hospitalisation à domicile* (HAD) schemes described in chapter 5. British experiment has relied largely on vague concepts of mutual goodwill and co-ordination between hospital and community staffs, or else exclusively on community resources. Inevitably under such arrangements, families of the sick bear weights of responsibilities for which they are often physically and psychologically ill equipped.

Through sensitive application of stringent assessment procedures prior to accepting their cases, French HAD schemes ensure that only hospitalised patients who want home care and whose families want them at home are admitted to their services. These and other conditions of acceptance, directed towards family protection rather than the convenience of hospital administrations and medical staffs, engender a spirit of co-operation between family and scheme which is a prerequisite to successful case management. This applies even in the absence of family members able to make any concrete contribution towards the patient's care. Conventions agreed annually between French hospital services and their financing mechanisms ensure that only genuine 'general hospital type' patients shall gain admission to a potentially costly amenity like HAD.

The NHS, which provides medical services universally free at the time of need, would similarly have to establish which patients might be entitled to integrated comprehensive home care such as is described in this volume before contemplating organisational arrangements for its delivery. First, towards this end, attempts have had to be made to conceptualise respective 'patient' groups according to estimated needs of their members and facilities necessary to meet these needs. After much deliberation (bearing in mind that, fit or ill, we are all regarded as the 'list patients' of some GP or another), it was agreed that the category of patients who might be offered options between hospital admission and a 'hospital at home'-type service must be 'full-time' or 'fully dependent' – such patients being incapable, literally in person or from their own domestic resources, of self-care. By such definition patients who, although perhaps partially incapacitated, could nevertheless look after themselves could be excluded.[1]

Next, local experiment would have to be introduced to test out requirements for the satisfaction of these patients' needs.

In 1977 enthusiastic support for 'hospital at home' (HAH) ideas from numerous doctors, health administrators, nurses, paramedical workers and voluntary organisations of patient concern led the Sainsbury Family Charitable Trusts to offer £200 000 to a health authority willing to conduct a three-year pilot scheme to test out the possibilities of a home care service based on the French experience. There were many contenders for the offer, but most based their proposals on geriatric need alone. These had to be eliminated from competition since a general hospital alternative, covering all age groups, was required. Of proposals satisfying this criterion it was virtually impossible to select one scheme put forward as being more suitable for testing purposes than another. Would it be better to opt for an inner city area, or one less complex in its health problems? In reality it would not much matter, since it was largely basic organisation and the capacity of a scheme to respond to local needs whatever they might be which would be put to the test. In the event Peterborough Health District of the Cambridgeshire Area Health Authority (Teaching) (now Peterborough Health Authority) was selected to undertake the experiment, conditional upon its willingness to continue the project as a permanent part of its amenities, subject to its being judged a success according to predetermined criteria.

Aims, organisation and programme

Members of the steering group set up to determine criteria for the launching and operation of the Peterborough experiment and to pilot the scheme through its various phases were agreed as follows:

(a) From Cambridgeshire AHA(T): a member of the authority; a member of the area team of Officers; all members of the Peterborough District Management Team; a consultant nominated by the Medical Executive Committee and a GP nominated by the Local Medical Committee

(b) Two officers of the Sainsbury Family Charitable Trusts

(c) A professor of community medicine from St George's Hospital Medical School, London

(d) The Director of the Domiciliary Health Care Unit, Brunel Institute of Social and Organisational Studies.

In April 1978 the steering group produced a document laying down criteria for the scheme entitled, 'Aims, organisation, and programme of the "Hospital-at-Home" pilot scheme in Peterborough Health District 1978–1981'.[2] This was intended to provide a frame of reference for the parties listed above and for those acting on their behalf. Its status, therefore, was that of an agreement among all concerned about their several responsibilities and an outline of the programme of the service. It confirmed steering group agreement on the following matters: the aims of the pilot scheme; the constitution and functions of the steering group; an outline of the service and its organisation; the nature of associated research activities; an outline of the programme of service and research activities; and financial arrangements.

The pilot scheme was agreed by the group to have two distinct though congruent aims:

(1) To set up, operate and test, between 1 April 1978 and 31 March 1981, the provision of health services for 'full-time' patients, by making such services available to them in their homes, provided that the following conditions were met: (i) that in-hospital treatment was not stipulated by the patient's doctor(s); (ii) that the assessor (see page 122) and co-ordinator (see page 122) of the service agreed that the patient's psychological, social and physical circumstances were suitable; (iii) that patient and family respectively did positively wish for domiciliary care – that is, they chose it in preference to hospital admission, this being a choice open to them.

(2) To carry out investigation of the scheme in order to increase explicit understanding of (i) concepts and principles relevant to domiciliary health care in particular and to health services in general; (ii) the standards of care available under the conditions of the pilot scheme, relative to other current comparable schemes, such as in-hospital care.

Responsibility for seeing that these aims were pursued rested with the steering group, from whom unanimity voting was required. Fulfilment of this responsibility required that there should be close contact between the group and staff working in the scheme, both in service and in research capacities. Such staff therefore might regularly attend steering group meetings and were likely to interact considerably with certain members of the group in their individual capacities. It fell to the steering group to ensure that the aims of the scheme were pursued in accordance with the intentions of all concerned. In particular, this related to the fundamental character of the scheme as an alternative to hospital care, allowing patients the choice of locus of care whenever medically and practically possible. The group had the early task of formulating criteria by which success or otherwise of the scheme might be judged.

It was agreed that, on the service side, the scheme would provide basic nursing (including general 'looking after') through its staff of nurses and aides, who, between them, and in appropriate combination with the patient's household, would be able to ensure for the patient that the necessary work would be done to guarantee his or her activities of daily living, as well as nursing prescribed by medical staff. It would also provide specialist work such as, for example, physiotherapy from its own staff or by arrangement with existing district resources, or from other agencies. Ultimate responsibility for services to patients would rest with the AHA, through an assessor and co-ordinator who would be appointees of the AHA and accountable to the District Administrator (assessor) and District Nursing Officer (co-ordinator) respectively. Nurses and aides would be organised under the co-ordinator (a nursing officer) who would also be responsible for equipment, materials, transport and records arrangements. Research requirements would be met through Brunel Institute's Domiciliary Health Care Unit and St George's Hospital Department of Community Medicine. The Sainsbury Trustees agreed to meet running and research costs up to a maximum of £204 000 over three years. The AHA agreed to cover costs of equipment and materials, staff transport and administrative expenses up to an agreed maximum of £23 000 plus an initial £5000 for capital equipment.

Peterborough is designated an expanding town in the throes of increasing its population by 100 000. Already its health district caters for nearly 200 000, including people living in isolated fenland areas where access is often difficult. A new hospital is scheduled for 1987, but until this has been built a serious shortage of hospital beds will continue. Recognising that the HAH services per patient would have to be on a far greater scale than those provided by primary care teams, Peterborough Health District had to decide whether to spread the activities of HAH over a large area or to concentrate them in one small locality. It chose the latter – a catchment area of 23 000 population served by three group and one single-handed practices – a total of 12 GPs.[3]

It is only when an attempt is made to put a novel idea into practice that one fully appreciates the strength of resistance on the one hand, and support on the other, to plans which might lead to disturbance, however small, in traditional ways of working. Primary care in Peterborough is better than that provided in most areas of my acquaintance. Some of its community nurses were already well satisfied with existing organisational arrangements for the care of the sick at home, wishing only for more staff and better resources. But others saw immediately the rationale of making special organisational arrangements for those amongst their patients who required guarantees of full-time care if they were to avoid hospital admission. Consequently, HAH ideas were met with suspicion and resentment amongst a few community nurses, although the attitudes of the majority ranged from cautious interest to enthusiastic and energetic support.

By and large hospital staffs liked our ideas, some, perhaps, because they opened up prospects of divesting beds of long-stay cases. But they thought us over-optimistic in our hopes of overcoming age-old problems of existing community provision, finding it difficult to visualise any system capable of covering all patient needs outside hospitals. Furthermore, they were rightly sceptical about the value, in terms of relieving hospital beds, of a scheme covering only a very small part of their total hospital catchment area.

Paramedical workers in Peterborough hospital were highly

cognisant of the need to extend their services to patients at home; recognising that rehabilitation, dietary regulation and disabled living assistance exclusively in a hospital setting frequently fails to equip the patient adequately for eventual discharge. Even so, some were sceptical about a scheme whereby much of their work might be undertaken by aides lacking professional qualification, albeit under their instruction and supervision.

Enthusiastic as they were about HAH ideas, being employed by local government (not by the health authority), hospital social workers could not participate in the Peterborough scheme as members integral to its organisation. The most they might hope for would be secondment from the Cambridgeshire County Council SSD, with freedom to devote their time and organise their work according to criteria and operational arrangements laid down by the scheme's steering group and assured through health authority management.

During the months of preparation prior to the appointment of an operational staff, the nursing co-ordinator of HAH, Peterborough, and the present author as its consultant/assessor had sought to gain professional and lay understanding of the concepts governing the scheme and the kind of organisation we thought would be necessary for its success. Now we had to concentrate on staff recruitment, induction and training; head-quarters preparation; assembly of essential equipment and materials; transport arrangements for their home delivery; and arrangements for patients' hospital attendances for tests and treatments which could not take place in their homes. Our earlier efforts to secure local understanding of HAH concepts and aims stood us in good stead in the practicalities of these tasks. Consequently, many potential problems stemming from lack of sound organisation in our service were minimised through personal goodwill and wishes for our success. We determined to follow as far as possible industrial relations' procedures with unions, for example, in portering, transport and HQ upkeep. Our earlier consultations with them in the planning stages of our work greatly eased this. Their members also appreciated that the scheme might bring benefits to themselves and their families in cases of sickness in the home. They saw for themselves need for flexibility in ways of working which would not be conceivable in their ordinary hospital duties.

Operational preparation

Prior to its creation in April 1978, little local preparation for the launching of the Peterborough scheme had taken place. Until the steering group had announced its aims, organisation and programme, no one really knew what to prepare for; added to which, the machinery by which new health initiatives are usually set in motion could not be applied because these had to be exercised *either* under hospital *or* under community health sector administration, whereas the HAH concept relied essentially on the welding together of the two sectors. The District Management Team (DMT) therefore had to create new administrative machinery unique to the scheme before the latter could become operational. Even then this machinery would not be in a position to mobilise personnel and resources in ways fully reflecting principles of integrated hospital/community care. Clearly, HAH Peterborough would have to rely by and large on liaisive and co-ordinative measures, based on personal qualities of goodwill and co-operation, without the organisational strength considered by French HAD schemes crucial to their success. In this respect it would resemble other recent home care experiments in Britain.

Preliminary talks with hospital consultants on the one hand and GPs on the other showed that most appreciated the benefits HAH might bring to their patients. When it came to attempting organisational arrangements aimed at making specialist services available outside hospital, however, only a minority of the GPs likely to be affected directly by the Peterborough scheme indicated willingness for formal change in their existing ways of working. This would inhibit the extent to which the DHA could allocate resources for HAH operation.

Although district nurses working in the locality of the scheme were reassured that district nursing qualifications would be required for all its home nurses (and hence there would be no question of hospital nurses stepping into roles traditionally played by themselves), some were antagonistic to any suggestion of possible change in their existing ways of working. Their voice and that of some GPs resistant to change made impossible the achievement of HAH Peterborough as a hospital/community integrated service. Nevertheless, convinced of the need to find ways of bringing together hospital and community sectors towards integrated ways of working, the health authority made tentative administrative arrangements to facilitate enhanced resource allocations in cases where individual GPs were prepared to countenance increased administrative intervention in the (non-clinical) management of such cases. Towards this end it placed HAH in the hands of *district* nursing and general administration, thereby spanning hospital and community divisions. This, at least, would provide for the control and monitoring of such hospital-held resources as were agreed by individual GPs to be requisite to their patients' proper care under HAH.

District administration would also provide for allocations of paramedical services, for which existing community health sectors of the NHS make no provision. It would also facilitate social worker support, in that social workers employed by local government are seconded to health districts and not to community health divisions. It would not, of course, resolve problems of principle, which require social worker support *integral to* HAH.

Staff appointments: nurses and patients' aides

The most pressing need now was for the appointment of operational staff: nurses responsible for cases placed in their care, and aides who would look after patients under the instruction and supervision of these nurses. Both kinds of appointment required the drawing up of job descriptions including elements outside traditional nursing responsibilities. Nurses would have to ensure that their changes were properly 'looked after', in addition to being provided with 'items' of nursing. Aides would have to perform tasks not attributable to nursing, as well as those that were, and hence the nurses to whom they were accountable would have to exercise skills and judgements outside *their* traditional expertise.

First, we had to find a title for these aides. We had to get away from the idea prevalent in community nursing that auxiliaries visiting the homes of patients under nursing supervision are responsible only for items of nursing, such as bathing and attending to toilet needs. Our aides were being appointed to help patients in any way they might need. At the suggestion of the District Nursing Officer, we decided to call them 'patients' aides', whereby they would supplement, or replace altogether, willing and competent support from members of the patient's family.[4]

Having drawn up job descriptions for HAH nurses and patients' aides, we were able to proceed with nursing appointments and inductions and selection and training of patients' aides. Nurses would have to learn to delegate much of their work, whereas they had been accustomed, and had enjoyed, working largely in isolation. In the drawing up of individual care programmes, according to which they would organise their own activities and those of patients' aides allocated to particular cases, they would have to take into account basic domestic and social needs as well as those of nursing. In fact, they would play roles similar to those of ward sisters in hospitals, with the added problems and possibilities of integrating family help with that of HAH personnel and the difficulties of ensuring medically prescribed services outside a hospital environment. They would not, like ward sisters, be able to take for granted arrangements for cooking, laundry and deliveries of essential supplies.

We wanted the people of Peterborough to regard HAH as an amenity potentially open to them if *they* wished to use it, not only if their doctors *selected* their cases for it. So far, all they had learned about the scheme was from sometimes inaccurate press and radio reports giving the impression it was a device to reduce demands on hospital beds and that it was essentially a scheme for the elderly. Alongside our staff recruitment campaign, and after consulting with the local Community Health Council, we spread our ideas to organisations such as the Women's Royal Voluntary Service, Mothers' Unions, Townswomen's Guilds, Senior Citizens' Clubs, and clubs for the deaf, blind and other disabled population groups: anywhere, in fact, where patients with problems of daily living and persons committed to helping them were likely to come together.

This approach led to a surge of public interest in HAH. Our advertisement for patients' aides attracted 150 applications (at a time of full employment in the area) for the equivalent of eight full-time posts. So many applicants seemed emminently suited to the work we had in mind for them, it was virtually impossible to be sure we selected the best. Some unsuccessful candidates said they would like to work for the scheme in a voluntary capacity, while the organisations we had approached with a view to getting our aims properly understood were enthusiastic about prospects of forming a volunteer corps around the scheme.

In the event, four posts were filled with full-time, permanent, staff. The remaining four posts were filled through a 'bank' of 30 aides, to be called upon in rotation, according to case requirements and at times suited to their own convenience.

Case records

With the nursing co-ordinator and two of the four nursing sister posts filled, training of patients' aides could now go ahead. We could not admit patients to our scheme until we had devised a case record system covering aspects of patient need as comprehensive as those of hospital patients; in addition, there had to be records of basic support provision, unnecessary in hospital case notes, since the basic requirements of hospitalised patients are automatically met through services divisions. It was also essential that we should include social worker and (where applicable) paramedical worker assessments and records of activities. Furthermore, provision would have to be made for the inclusion of relevant observations from responsible members of patients' own entourages. As the HAH personnel in closest continuing touch, patients' aides would provide valuable evidence as to general case progress.

We had to avoid situations whereby medical records on HAH patients might be maintained simultaneously but separately and without co-ordination in GP surgeries and/or hospital outpatients' departments as well as in HAH files' and whereby patients might simultaneously receive drugs and other items of treatment from both these sources, unbeknown to HAH personnel. We had to make recording provision for programmes of treatment and care continuous upon those of prior hospitalisation, despite the fact that we would have no powers to ensure this, it being contingent upon GPs to determine for themselves whether or not they would pursue hospital-originated programmes. Likewise, we had no authority to insist that GPs attending HAH patients should make their observations in HAH records. All we could do would be to devise the system we thought to be most fool-proof in the circumstances and to hope that individual GPs would recognise it to be in the best interests of their patients.

We recognised, in principle, the rights of patients to hold their own dossiers. (Doctors themselves would, of course, decide where essentially clinical records would be lodged.) Hence, we determined that, as far as we could judge, it would not be harmful to the interests of the patient in a particular case for these dossiers to be placed in the custody of a responsible relative, subject to the wishes of the patient. But many of our patients would not be in fit conditions to state their wishes. Some might be cared for by neighbours to whom they would not wish to disclose confidences. Our system had to take account of all these factors.

The system we ultimately devised was held by all concerned to be a radical advance on any known case record format for non-hospitalised patients. The dossier would be maintained in two sections – an HQ file and a bedside file. The HQ file would be available to GPs, hospital doctors and other professionals, and would include information considered by any of these professionals unsuitable for inclusion in the bedside file. The latter would be placed in a robust, brightly coloured, cleanable, ring file, reusable for subsequent patients. It would be divided into four sections: medical (including prescription sheets); nursing; paramedical; social. It would include instruction sheets for patients' aides and provision for their day-to-day recordings of developments in the case, to which caring relatives might contribute. Clear instructions at the front cover would advise families what to do in an emergency and what HAH could and could not do for its patients. A see-through plastic envelope, containing, for example, blood group, diabetic and anticoagulant cards, usually to be found in pockets, wallets or drawers, would be secured at the front of the file. Spare sheets of writing paper, carbon and envelopes would be inserted at the back; and a ball-point pen would be secured on a cord tied to the ring file so that visiting personnel would always have something to hand with which to write.

On the patient's discharge from HAH, HQ and bedside files would be amalgamated. If the patient had to be re-admitted to hospital, the record would accompany him/her. On discharge or death it would be filed in the district hospital medical records department (having previously been registered with a hospital case number). GPs would be able to write their own case summaries for inclusion in their surgery records in ways similar to those written by hospital doctors to GPs on a patient's discharge from hospital.

Pharmacy

Prescription arrangements for HAH Peterborough patients stimulated more debate among members of the local Family Practitioners' Committee (FPC) than did any other single element. We had originally assumed that there would be no problem about the supply of drugs. Since we were providing a parallel service to general hospital admission, our patients would receive drugs free of charge, just as do hospital patients. We had discussed this with area and district pharmacists, who readily accepted the notion in principle. Some GPs were ready to modify their traditional prescribing habits accordingly. But the weight of FPC opinion was against it. HAH patients must obtain their drugs from the high street shops, like other GP patients. The implications of this ruling went beyond those of payment. We had assumed that we would be able to exercise a measure of control over drugs by reason of their being HAH property. As patients' property their regulation by HAH nurses would have to rely on the willingness of individual GPs to observe the guidelines suggested for their participation in HAH activities and the abilities of individual HAH nurses to persuade patients and their families to observe recommendations for safe drug regulation. To aid in the latter's safe-keeping we bought lock-up metal boxes for use where patients had no secure storage facilities of their own.

Modifications and findings

In final preparation for the admission of our first patients in October 1978, Peterborough Health District circulated for distribution, through local GPs and hospital doctors, an advice and information booklet for prospective patients and their families. To the concern of many involved in the setting up and operation of the pilot scheme, we had not managed to obtain firm rulings that, should an HAH admission prove unsatisfactory for medical, nursing or social reasons, the alternative of general hospital admission would be assured. GPs were of the opinion that, in the event of a breakdown in HAH arrangements, they would be able to obtain a hospital bed for a patient without difficulty.

After five months uneasy operation in its initial form, it was clear that the Peterborough experiment had been based on too small a catchment area to provide, in numbers and varieties, hospital cases necessary for it to prove its worth as a district hospital parallel. Although, case for case, hospital staffs where involved were highly satisfied both with its approach and its provisions, numbers of their patients affected were negligible, compared with the district hospital population as a whole. Furthermore, it was apparent from only 32 GP referrals (of which only 25 cases had been judged by HAH personnel suitable cases for admission) that either local GPs were having difficulty in finding suitable cases, or else they were holding back from using the scheme in its existing form. When referrals began to show a downward trend the steering group had to act swiftly to avert what seemed to be its pending collapse.

Two major changes were made: one constitutional and the other extending the scheme's catchment area to cover the whole of Peterborough. The latter alone may well have been sufficient to set it on the upward trend again. But major administrative problems of integrating hospital and community elements of its make-up had not been resolved, nor did it seem possible that they could be. GP opposition to any organisational arrangement providing for greater hospital involvement in domiciliary patient care than is traditional persisted.

In modifying administrative arrangements for the second phase of HAH Peterborough its steering group did not envisage radical change in its ultimate aims. Although now under community nursing management, it was incapable of ensuring integrated hospital/community operation; at least it retained the capacity to enhance primary care services with varieties and levels of services presently denied to them. Although there could be no guarantee that these would be fully utilised and deployed with optimum effectiveness, they could hardly fail but to bring advantages to many Peterborough patients hitherto of necessity hospitalised.

Fortunately for the steadily increasing flow of patients admitted to the scheme in its second phase (now drawn from the whole of the district hospital catchment area instead of one small locality), HAH had managed to prove during its first phase the rationale of its original criteria for operation designed to protect the interests of patients and their families. It continued to develop concepts of patient support through the training and formation of its patients' aides. But, unhappily, now being exclusively a community nursing service, hopes of paramedical participation in the scheme could no longer be fully realised. For example, the original practice of including therapists in the training of newly appointed patients' aides was abandoned and there was under-utilisation of the time and skills of these therapists, allocated for HAH activities. When, under its second phase, integral social worker support for the scheme was abandoned, its nurses identified very little in the way of social services requirements among their charges.[5]

Organisational modifications to HAH Peterborough (Mark 2) were accompanied by those of research requirements, responsibility for which was now passed from outside the health authority to internal provision.[6]

Costs of the Peterborough experiment were high: on average almost equal, per patient-day, to the estimated cost of financing a case in a bed of the district hospital. This is not surprising, as the Peterborough scheme in its final form was structurally incapable of exercising the kinds of controls necessary to modify costs according to annual budgets available for its day-to-day operation. It was not required to produce, as in the cases of the various *hospitalisation à domicile* schemes in France, evidence of costs per patient day on average less than half of those of the district hospitals in whose catchment areas they were situated. But it is difficult to make valid costs comparisons between home and hospital care; so many variables are involved. This is borne out by the findings of other researchers in the field. Readers might like to study these by reference to the numerous publications on the subject listed in appendix A (see pages 195–6).

Despite its relatively-high cost and other problems, the Peterborough experiment was judged so highly in terms of patient benefit that it has now been adopted by the Peterborough Health Authority as a permanent part of its amenities. Does it really matter that it is now regarded as an extension of primary, rather than a new concept of secondary, care? The answer must be 'yes', because, although patients whom it is intended to benefit are uniquely those suffering major (including terminal) disabling illness, it cannot as a primary care service guarantee firm lines of accountability and responsibility to and from the DHA for the medical services it seeks to provide; specialist, paramedical, social work and basic support services commensurate with patients' pre-assessed needs; maintenance of nursing services at levels and of varieties pre-assessed to be the minimum necessary; identification and mobilisation of willing family, neighbourhood and voluntary services available in particular cases; monitoring and maintenance of such services in accordance with day-to-day fluctuations in patients conditions; or that patients themselves, with the agreement of their caring relatives, will be afforded genuine options between HAH and hospital admission. Furthermore, it does not now have the administrative capacity to ensure its own optimum effective, economic operation.

Despite uncertainty about the organisational strength and potential of HAH Peterborough, there can be no doubt about the status it has achieved in the eyes of the local people. A measure of this can be gained from the fact that a Friends Group, set up in May 1981, has already (mid-1983) donated over £23 000 to the DHA towards further HAH activities.[7] The significance of this cannot be judged in monetary terms alone. It is a mark of the extent to which local people will come together in support of statutory activities when they are seen to give priority consideration to the aspirations of patients themselves.

References

(1) Cang, S. and Clarke, F., 'Home care of the sick – an emerging general analysis based on schemes in France', *Community Health*, 1978, **9** (3), 167–71; Cang, S., '"Full-time" and "part-time" patients: an analysis of patient needs and their implications for domiciliary and institutional care', in *Health Services* (E. Jaques, ed.), Heinemann Educational, London, 1978, chapter 11.

(2) 'Aims, organisation, and programme of the "Hospital-at-Home" pilot scheme in Peterborough Health District 1978–1981', unpublished document, Cambridgeshire Area Health Authority (Teaching), Cambridge, 1978.

(3) 'Proposed hospital at home scheme', unpublished document, Cambridgeshire Area Health Authority (Teaching), Cambridge, 1978.

(4) Minutes of the HAH Steering Group meeting of 17 May 1978, Cambridgeshire Area Health Authority (Teaching), Cambridge.

(5) 'Hospital at Home, Peterborough: the pilot scheme, April 1978–March 1981', unpublished report, Peterborough Health Authority, Peterborough, 1983.

(6) *Ibid.*

(7) *Ibid.*

8 'Hospital at home' and the medical profession

In principle the mainstream of medical opinion in Britain favours an integrated health system. But there is considerable doubt within the profession about its ability to achieve it and many doctors are opposed to the organisational measures which would favour its introduction.

Patients suffer the ill effects of divisive medical policies, particularly when they are in too weak a state themselves to co-ordinate the various elements of their care and treatment. Prevailing attitudes on the part of both profession and public are that, despite its weaknesses, existing NHS organisation is by and large satisfactory. Are indications to the contrary sufficient to justify the claim of this book that organisational change is crucial to more effective mobilisation of curative and caring skills than at present appears possible?

Doctors are organised in a fashion which reduces contributions they might make towards both prevention and cure of illness. Hospital admissions often have nothing to do with need for specialist care or use of hospital equipment. Failure to make hospital referrals frequently results in inaccurate diagnosis and inappropriate or improperly supervised treatment. Some patients suffer rather than benefit from the consequences of hospital admissions.

Hospital doctors decry waste of hospital beds and other amenities; GPs, deprivation of proper facilities for the home care of their patients. Seldom do members of either group ask themselves, 'What of the dilemma for the patient who requires specialist and/or comprehensive care but neither wishes nor essentially requires hospitalisation?'

Medical provision in the NHS is founded on concepts of primary care in the community, secondary care in hospitals. Lest readers might think my view, that primary health care teams should not be responsible for looking after fully dependent patients, is ill founded, I would point to findings of research analyses conducted by doctors themselves which suggest serious shortcomings in the general practices upon which these primary health care teams are based.

In July 1978 *The Sunday Times* published in consecutive issues a two-part summary of a searching enquiry into what appeared to be the beginnings of a crisis in the NHS.[1] It drew its evidence of this from various professional and government studies ranging from those of a clinical kind to those mainly concerned with health politics and administration. It demonstrated the irrationality inherent in a service in which professional independence is maintained even when it results in gross contrasts of treatment. It found that clinical judgement so intensively individual bears unsatisfactorily on many patients.

The enquiry found that both members of patients admitted to hospitals and their lengths of stay increased according to numbers of beds available, yet waiting lists did not significantly decline; the conclusion being that sickness expands to fill the number of beds available. It reported that in 1976, Dr David Owen, then Minister of State at the Department of Health, pointed to disparities of clinical freedom, giving doctors the right to say how long patients should stay in hospital. For example, some consultants kept peptic ulcer cases in hospital for six days, others for 26 days; some kept hernia cases for two days, others for 12 days; appendicectomy cases, three days as opposed to 10 days; tonsillectomy cases, one day as opposed to five days; hysterectomy cases, three days as opposed to 36 days. Owen also pointed to a study of six hospitals showing that, in one, 26 per cent of male patients suffering tuberculosis were kept in hospital for a year; while, in another, all were discharged within 90 days. In no cases were shorter stays found to have any adverse effects on the patients.

The enquiry then went on to demonstrate the meaning of clinical freedom amongst GPs by examining patient referral rates to hospital specialists. It pointed to a study covering four practices which found that these varied from five per thousand in one practice to 115 per thousand in another; from six per thousand in a third, to 256 per thousand in a fourth. The researchers could find no clinical explanations for these variations. One possible reason was given as financial. Since under the NHS GPs are paid so much per list patient per annum, the more people on the doctor's list the greater the income and the less the time that can be spent on each patient. If pressure on time becomes too great, there may be a tendency to refer all but the simplest cases to specialists. Another sample study, the enquiry stated, found that some GPs prescribed drugs from four to ten times more frequently than others.

All doctors, specialists and GPs alike, go through common selection procedures when embarking on their careers, and candidates selected receive a common basic training. In terms of basic qualification there has been no difference between specialists and GPs for well over a century. Most doctors take up medicine because they are interested in healing rather than in the prevention in disease. Some doctors opt to be GPs because they have a special interest in disease prevention, but perhaps more seek GP appointments for domestic and family reasons or because they feel they have little prospect of professional advancement through the mainstream of hospital medicine. Inevitably the reasons which lead doctors to take up general practice must, to a certain extent, determine the kind of service they provide to the public.

No-one knows how good a service GPs provide because there is no means of assessing it accurately. But there is broad agreement within the medical profession that standards are low in many respects. Reports of hasty examinations, inadequate screenings, inefficient diagnoses, negligence in midwifery and careless prescriptions occur too frequently to be ignored.

In 1972, in an attempt to gain further insight into what happens between GPs and their patients when the latter present symptoms of illness, the Department of Health and Social Security (DHSS) commissioned a research programme to be carried out by the Department of General Practice at Manchester University. [2] It was agreed that there should be a two-and-a-half-year look at doctors in their surgeries, on their rounds and, where possible, at patients' bedsides. The purpose was to try to discover if there were features common to all consultations and whether there were any features of the latter which could be described as doctor-centred idiosyncracies. Parallel with this there was to be a programme aimed at training potential GP-trainers and enabling the research team to gain insights into new methods of training developed in the previous 20 years.

Part of the study was centred on the findings of 60 UK, five Dutch and six Irish GPs, who volunteered scrutiny of tape-recorded consultations with nearly 2500 patients. This found that most GPs worked within a frame of reference which required both illnesses and patients to fit a pre-judged pattern, connected with the ways in which doctors learn to cope with diagnosing organic illness. They had 'few sociological tools of analysis to support their organic diagnostic tools'.[4] The study confirmed previously held views that the majority of doctors will find ways of practising the kinds of medicine for which they were trained.

An analysis of general practice made in 1960[5] divides the therapeutic behaviour of doctors into four categories: advice, explanation, discussion and listening. It points to evidence in the field of communication studies that most listening is selective and suggests that doctors are as selective as any other population group. Yet there is little evidence that listening as such is an integral part of medical training – if it is taught it is always as a function of something else. Seemingly, those doctors who can and do conduct analyses based on sympathetic listening do so in spite of, rather than because of, their medical training.[6]

In the findings published in 1976 of the enquiry commissioned by the DHSS, Byrne and Long[7] make their point by quoting from *The Future General Practitioner*[8] an extreme example of a doctor who works through a rigid frame of reference:

'The doctor may insist on focusing on certain aspects of the patient's problem because they are the easiest for him to handle. He will then refuse to allow the patient to tell him anything else, or refuse to hear. To obtain his greatest satisfaction the doctor usually wants to find a patient with a serious acute illness that has interesting features – elicited and recognised by him with great acumen – and one who responds rapidly, completely and gratefully to proper therapy.'

This statement was written by a group of doctors about doctors![9]

Few people, doctors included, would deny that there has been a drop in public confidence in the medical profession in recent years.[10] There is ample reason for public concern about standards of medical care. The BMA suggests that hospital patients may be in danger because junior hospital doctors are dropping with fatigue.[11] The number of home visits by GPs was nearly halved between 1969 and 1978.[12] In Britain's big cities the chances are that an attempt to contact a GP will fail. The doctor who eventually comes to the house is likely to be a stranger, who can only guess at the contents of the patient's medical file locked away in the GP's surgery. Deputising services are now used by about 10 500 of the country's 25 000 GPs. In London and some other cities, 90 per cent of doctors use them to varying degrees. A survey of London doctors has shown that if you ring your GP there is a 56 per cent chance of talking to an answering machine, rather than to a GP or receptionist.[13]

Serious as is the crisis of confidence in our hospitals, it must be viewed in a rather different light from that in GPs. Health authorities have clearly defined responsibilities for hospitalised patients. It is to be hoped that they have resources at their disposal to look after the latter while they are being treated, and ward nursing staff who have responsibilities to identify and act upon patient needs outside the clinical field. The fact that doctors may not listen to their patients may not be so important in hospitals, where other staff also have a duty to listen, as in a GP's surgeries, where only the doctor may be present.

It has never been made clear what responsibilities GPs have, other than those of a strictly clinical nature and which can be met by prescription. Some GPs make sure their patients have every support service they can lay their hands on. Others would not think to question families about how they were coping with sick members.

The findings of the 1976 study on doctor–patient relationships are of significant importance in considering the provision of domiciliary alternatives to hospital care: additionally so in view of the double standards which the NHS applies to hospital versus community care. Are we wise, even, to contemplate services which would enable more patients to stay at home when we know that, under existing health organisation, those patients could not be guaranteed the support they may need?

Compared with pre-NHS days, GPs can now *do* far more things to help their patients and are consequently more likely to

be judged on their peformances. Pressure to keep up with the
latest technological advances and medical discoveries, and to be
aware of possible iatrogenic consequences of the latter, imply an
essential need for modern GPs to have access to hospital resources
currently denied to them or difficult in access. Dual expectations
of them in both prevention and cure are exacting. At the same
time their own high relative autonomy and inadequate public
knowledge as to what actually goes on in general practice, plus
resistance to. medical audit, present a dilemma for those responsible for health standards under the NHS. Should and could
GPs be drawn into the mainstream of pathological medicine
relying on hospital services? If so, what arrangements should be
made for the development of preventive health services?

The need for integrated specialist/GP services in domiciliary care

A marked increase in medical specialisation and a sharp drop in
the numbers of GPs who regard home visits as part of their
routine duties raise great concern for the well-being of patients
who do not have hospital links and who cannot get to their GPs'
surgeries. It is not realistic to expect doctors, GP or hospital, to
develop home-visiting medical services under existing circumstances. Doctors trained to treat patients in institutions find that
meeting patients in their own homes creates uneasiness and
decreases professional self-confidence. Furthermore, there are
physical hazards in working in isolation from colleagues and
outside institutional protection. These hazards (which apply to
all professional groups brought into physical contact with their
clients) present a particular threat to GPs who undertake
responsibility for cases which should, it could be held, have been
referred to hospital.

There are some valid reasons why it might not be feasible or
desirable to develop domiciliary specialist provision at the
expense of the hospital sector. Home visiting is costly in terms of
time and money. When patients are hospitalised they are readily
available whenever consultants might wish to examine them. In

terms of public benefit at large, a consultant's time spent on seeing one patient at home might be more profitably spent in seeing a number of patients in hospital. If it can be demonstrated, however, that certain patients get better more quickly or do not get so ill in the first place when they are nursed at home, their need for prolonged specialist attention is reduced.

In 1976, Professor P. Nixon, cardiologist at Charing Cross Hospital observed:

'Hospital care and investigation can be alarming, and the arousal caused by an admission can precipitate a breakdown in those who are too ill to accommodate to a change of habits . . . . All [coronary patients] must learn to avoid sleep deprivation . . . . When a patient leaves hospital after a coronary breakdown, he goes home in the phase of ill-health with many more problems than he had at the point of breakdown. The physical and emotional effects of being in hospital usually decondition and regress him and increase his arousal.'[14]

In 1982 he opened a home visiting service with the aim of reducing such incidence to a minimum.

It is axiomatic that the patients most likely to be upset by hospital routines are those who find it most distressing to leave their homes and families. The clinical freedom of doctors to determine where, as well as how, their patients should be treated is severely curtailed by institutionally orientated health systems. But since the medical profession itself largely determines health care patterns in Britain, it is part of the clinical responsibility of its members to make sure their patients do not suffer ill effects from hospital admissions which could be avoided. At its simplest, clinical freedom means that in medical matters only a doctor can make final decisions. This may appear reasonable, but clinical freedom based on a system whereby the only sure way of obtaining specialist attention may be to bypass the GP and gain direct access to hospital leaves the majority of the sick population dependent on GP services which, to say the least, are patchy in quality and quantity, according to where patients live and the respective abilities of the latter to attract medical attention. Perhaps specialists like Professor Nixon would welcome general hospital facilities enabling them to attend more of their patients in the relaxing environments of their homes.

Theoretically, the NHS enables every British subject to identify with a GP who knows his or her home and family background and who can therefore take these into account when determining treatment needs. However, only some GPs in some areas apply these principles of family doctoring to their work. The consequence is that a large section of the patient population is deprived of the medical services for which it pays and without which health may deteriorate. The medical profession knows this; but proposals from amongst its ranks for remedies usually stop short of solutions based on a fusion of community and hospital medical services. There may be important reasons of patient concern why such a fusion should not take place. If so this requires to be demonstrated.

In Britain, organised and critical questioning of medical practices by doctors themselves is almost unknown, while that from outside the profession does not always take account of the enormous burden of responsibility which the public at large is glad to place on the doorstep of the profession. In making a case for a realignment of medical services to provide for treatment in whichever environment, hospital or home, is most likely to benefit the patient, we have to bear in mind that wider patient options in decisions affecting health imply greater patient (and family) responsibility for decisions traditionally made by doctors *for* their patients.

Most health politicians, administrators and representatives of the lay public shrink from urging change in the NHS which would involve GP accountability to health authorities rather than their employment under independent contract to FPCs. Following the experiences of Aneuran Bevan when he attempted to introduce salaried GP services (see page 36), they appear to assume that such a move would result in a mass 'walk-out' by GPs and, in consequence, the collapse of the NHS.

We can never know what would have happened had Bevan pushed through his original proposals. But there are now indications, particularly among emerging doctors, many of whom will ultimately become GPs, that their accountability to health authorities is a necessary condition of their entitlement to facilities of the kinds they have enjoyed in their hospital appointments. While many GPs of the older generation, with thriving, unharassed, financially rewarding practices in sought-after localities, might cling to outdated concepts of individual freedoms, more and more of the younger generation would willingly forgo some of these for better access to resources than is presently conceivable, enabling them to treat and care for their patients more effectively than is presently possible. Given GP access to general hospital beds, it is likely that their numbers would multiply.

With these thoughts in mind I have concluded that a service like 'hospital at home' would be welcomed by all doctors who place their patients' interests before those of personal advancement.

References

(1) 'Inquiry into the NHS: Part II. The high price of letting the doctors decide', *The Sunday Times*, 23 July 1978.
(2) Byrne, P. S., and Long, B. E., *Doctors Talking to Patients*, HMSO, London, 1976.
(3) *Ibid.*, p. 8.
(4) *Ibid.*, p. 8.
(5) *Ibid.*, p. 15. See also Scott, R., *et al.*, 'Just what the doctor ordered – an analysis of general practice', *British Medical Journal*, **ii**, 293–9, 1960.
(6) Byrne and Long, *op. cit.*, p. 15.
(7) *Ibid.*, p. 15.
(8) *Ibid.*, p. 14.
(9) *Ibid.*, p. 14.
(10) Widgery, D., *Health in Danger*, Macmillan, London, 1979.
(11) 'BMA press report', *The Guardian*, 19 April 1980.
(12) *Ibid.*; see figures prepared by Intercontinental Medical Statistics.
(13) 'Strangers take over as GPs take awaydays', *The Sunday Times*, 24 May 1981.
(14) Nixon, P. G. F., 'The human function curve with special reference to cardiological disorders', *The Practitioner*, 1976, **217**, 765 and 935.

9 Nurses and home care of the sick

As early as the beginning of the eighteenth century, doctors recognised their need for skilled auxiliaries to enable their own professional advancement. They found these auxiliaries in nurses, devoted to the care of the sick but without professional strengths of their own by which to raise their status beyond that of menial workers and skivvies. Thereafter nurses have had a battle on their hands to establish a professional identity not totally restricted by requirements on them from their medical colleagues.

Early medical fears that nurses might gain from their close contact with patients, at the expense of doctors interested more in the medical condition than the person, prompted these doctors to set rigid limits, beyond which nurses must not act in their administrations to the sick. A nurse, said one English physician of the past, laying down a set of qualifications for nurses, must be 'observant to follow the Physician's orders duly: not be so conceited of her own skills as to give her own medications privately'.[1] As physicians relied less and less on the laying on of hands and increasingly applied the knowledge and skills of modern scientific and technological discovery, it became more and more crucial to effective patient care that nurses should not take on the roles of doctors. To assume prescribing rights of their own would be to widen dangers of iatrogenic illness, whilst neglect of duties traditionally incorporated within their roles would deprive patients of the ever increasing levels and qualities of care which they require whilst undergoing potentially dangerous and debilitating treatments.

Modern nursing incorporates intensive care and sophisticated treatments as well as primary health care of an elementary kind. Basic qualification is not now sufficient to enable professional advancement in any direction. Hospital nurses have to undergo additional specialist training before they can be considered for senior appointments in management and in many units (for example, psychiatric, dermatological, surgical, cardiac). Community nurses must qualify in district nursing or health visiting before being allocated rounds of their own. As a broad rule, specialisation does not equip a nurse to work across the boundaries of hospital and community, exceptions being, for example, in psychiatry, mental after-care and geriatrics. As far as general nursing is concerned it is left to hospital and district nurses to co-ordinate their activities, as they individually think fit. Little monitoring goes on to establish the extent to which this occurs.

Domestic and housekeeping elements of patient care in hospitals, which prior to the demise if hospital matrons were traditional to roles of nursing, have now been hived off to non-nursing service divisions. Community nurses do not have to concern themselves with such matters because they are the responsibility of patients' families and/or local authority personal social departments. Nevertheless, concern about basic patient support is ever present in the mind of the conscientious community nurse.

It is hardly surprising that high levels of stress and anxiety are chronic among nurses. Many are acutely aware that their profession is in a serious state. They eagerly seek solutions and there have been many recent changes in expressed nursing aims and policies. Yet there is strong resistance to their implementation from within the profession and equally strong resistance to attempts at changes initiated from outside. Professional and public expectations add, sometimes intolerably, to the high personal standards which most nurses set for themselves.[2]

Where problems of hospital nursing seriously affect the work of doctors, the latter can usually be relied upon to press for solutions which nurses themselves are unable to achieve. For example, doctors have insisted on specially selected and trained nurses in their operating theatres and intensive care units; ward sisters no longer have to cope as they once did with nurse training as well as ward management and case responsibility. By and large hospital patients have benefitted from such moves. Does the same apply to the home-bound?

Seemingly, GPs are not in a position to act collectively towards improved domiciliary nursing provision – perhaps they are broadly satisfied with things as they are. Such action in this respect as does occur is usually undertaken by individual GPs exceptionally motivated in favour of home care. Few would favour moves leading to increased demand for domiciliary visits and night calls from patients enabled to stay in their own homes by reason of increased home nursing services.

Community nurses deeply concerned with the non-clinical needs of their charges lay themselves open to stresses and worries which they are seldom in positions to resolve. Some try to do so: by attending patients in their off-duty hours; enlisting volunteer help, which they are not in positions adequately to monitor; pressurising social services departments already over-committed to other urgent calls on their resources. In each case the patient is liable to feel an encumbrance on family friends and community nurse, obliged to resort to insitutional admissions in order to relieve loved ones of their worries and responsibilities.

In both hospital and community sectors of the NHS, staff and resource shortages are often held responsible for failures in patient care. Of course these shortages do cause lowered standards, but inefficient management may also be an important contributory factor, or even their main cause. In some areas staff:patient ratios are unduly high without evidence of patient benefit. Bad management may be responsible for bad nursing practice; excessive staff turnover; failure to train students adequately for their real future roles; and high levels of nurse anxiety and stress. These add to the stress on patients of illness and hospitalisation and have adverse effects on such factors as recovery rates. One investigation connects the latter directly with the morale of nursing staff: 'the social structure of nursing is defective not only as a means of handling anxiety, but also as a method of organising its tasks'.[3]

Defence systems found within the nursing profession.

' . . . prevent true insight into the nature of problems and realistic appreciation of their seriousness. Thus, only too often, no action can be taken until a crisis is very near or has actually occurred. This is the eventuality we fear in the British general hospital nursing services. Even if there is no acute crisis, there is undoubtedly a chronic state of reduced effectiveness, which in itself is serious enough.'[4]

Organisational reform

Growing concern about shortages of trained nurses and an apparent decline in the status of the profession led to the setting up in 1963, of a Government committee of inquiry, whose findings were published in what came to be known as the Salmon Report.[5] Concern was largely related to conditions in hospitals, where it was noted that the title 'matron' was applied equally to nursing heads of hospitals of all sizes and that there was no clear distinctions between their respective rights and duties. Furthermore, as men were increasingly joining the profession, the title 'ward sister' had become anachronistic. The Committee found that the role of nurses as administrators was poorly defined and that there was confusion over the relative status of general nursing, midwifery, psychiatric nursing and teaching. Salmon recommended that status should be determined by the kinds of decisions being made, not by the number of beds controlled or the type of patient nursed.[6]

In 1968 the Seebohm Report persuaded the Government that health visiting should lose its links with social work.[7] Accordingly, in 1970 the Council for Training Health Visitors, set up jointly in 1962 with the Central Council for the Education and Training of Social Workers, lost its links with the latter. When, following NHS reorganisation in 1974, health authorities lost their medical social workers to local authority social services departments, the Council for the Education and Training of Health Visitors, set up in 1970, extended its qualifications requirements to cover social work skills now lost to the NHS.

Also in 1968, the DHSS set up a working party to consider the extent to which Salmon proposals on nursing structures and salaries were applicable to community nursing services. Its findings were published in the Mayston Report of 1969 and commended to local authorities, who at the time were responsible for community services of the NHS.[8]

The report noted that health visitors were concerned with the health of the household as a whole, health education, the early detection of abnormalities in children, the school health service and general assistance to families in difficulties. Home nurses were recognised to provide skilled care under the direction of GPs in patients' homes and in health centres. The report recommended their attachment to general practices, concentrating on rehabilitation, elementary home physiotherapy and care of the elderly and chronic sick.

This wide interpretation of the role of community nurses led to conclusions of need for management structures similar to those applying in hospitals. The Mayston Report proposed that: every local authority should appoint a chief nursing officer; senior nursing staff structure should be reviewed immediately; three levels of managers should be appointed; management training should be introduced for senior community nurses. Qualified district nurses would hence become first line managers parallel to the charge-nurse/ward sister grade of the Salmon structure. The Report failed to consider to what extent community health divisions had powers or authority to pursue policies and command resources their managers would need in order properly to perform their respective management functions.

NHS reorganisation in 1974 consolidated, under central government, nursing reorganisation which had already taken place under local government following implementation of proposals of the Salmon and Mayston Reports. One important aim of this consolidation was to integrate hospital and community nursing services towards effective continuing care programmes for the sick. It was anticipated that this might be achieved, with minimum disturbance of recent nursing management changes in respective hospital and community sectors following the recommendations of Salmon and Mayston, through district level integration. Accordingly, the posts of chief nursing officer (hospital) and director of nursing services (community) were superseded by the single post of district nursing officer, over both hospital and community sectors.[9]

Running throughout organisational reforms in the NHS during the past two decades has been the notion that nurses must be relieved of 'non-nursing' duties. The extent to which nurses should concern themselves with the basic support of their charges (for example, nourishment, maintenance of sick-room standards of cleanliness and furnishings, patient comfort and psychological well-being commensurate with clinical requirements of the case) has never been formally established. The question did not arise in the days of hospital matrons, because they were responsible for virtually every aspect of patient care as well as the management of personnel (nurses, domestics, catering staffs and so on) employed in them.

The NHS Reorganisation Act of 1973 required the setting up by health authorities of service departments responsible for certain aspects of patient care hitherto the responsibility of now defunct hospital matrons (for example, domestic, laundry and catering departments). This meant that financial and status recognition for nursing management, achieved by Salmon, were accompanied by the dropping of management responsibilities now in the hands of non-nursing departments. At the same time similar community nursing management career structures achieved by Mayston required no evidence of commensuration with management responsibilities actually undertaken. Unlike hospital management, community nursing management is not, and never has been, concerned with elements of patient care classified as 'non-nursing'. It has not needed to be, since patients whose families cannot cope with their basic support have to be admitted to hospital.

Nursing reform of recent years in both hospital and community sectors of the NHS has often led to lowering of job satisfaction among practising nurses. Many in hospitals feel that management bears too heavily upon them to permit ways of working which they themselves feel to be in the best interests of their charges. While, in the community, GP practice-attached health visitors and district nurses are often faced with conflicts of management and expectations of them by GPs which prevent them from developing ways of working which they themselves feel best meet the needs of individual patients and their families. In any case, they do not have access to the resources they potentially need for this. Had doctors not been preoccupied with interprofessional interests, nurses absorbed with the creation of career grades in management, and social workers with achieving professional status independent of other health and welfare services, NHS reform of the past two decades might have resulted in great improvements in provisions for the sick both in and outside hospital. In the event, many, with justification, hold that no significant improvement has been achieved; indeed that, in many respects, nursing, like medical and social care, has deteriorated for reasons which cannot be attributed to lack of resources alone.

Progress, or lack of progress, in hospital nursing is related to causes fundamentally different from those which apply to community nursing. Health authorities are *wholly* responsible for hospital patients. Nurses are delegated responsibilities by these authorities to make sure individual patients are properly looked after in all respects. GPs, not accountable to health authorities, are responsible for patients outside hospitals. GP responsibilities are uniquely of a *clinical* kind. (It is up to each individual GP to decide the extent of his/her interest outside these.) They utilise their practice-attached nurses accordingly.

Thus, Mayston's proposals, based on concepts of practice-attachments for nurses concentrating on rehabilitation, elementary home physiotherapy and care of the elderly and chronic sick, were notional, rather than a realistic basis for organisational community nursing reform. The Salmon gradings as applied to community nursing were not necessarily a reflection of respective management responsibilities held in practice. What practice-attached nurses *do* for their charges depends primarily on what is expected of them by the GPs to whose practices they are attached and, secondly, on what resources are available to them in the course of their duties. Neither aspect suggests heavy management responsibilities on the part of the nursing administrators responsible for their work, other than those in connection with staff selection, training and allocation, and dealing with matters of arbitration as they arise. This is not to say there is no need for them. Indeed, where patients who are the subject of this book are concerned, skilled nursing management is perhaps the greatest single factor in case success.

Traditional comparative freedom from administrative and close monitoring control is deeply valued by today's community nurses. For many patients it works satisfactorily because it enables establishment of relaxed relationships between nurse and patient over months, perhaps years, of home visits of brief duration. Provided that such visits are all the patient requires, neither nurse nor patient suffer, on the one hand, a sense of having failed the patient or, on the other, consequences of neglect. Most district nurses, however, have on their case-loads at any given time at least one patient whom, they feel, ought to be in hospital because they cannot provide him/her with the requisite care. If the patient does not want to be in hospital, the nurse may gain great satisfaction from that one case because she has been largely instrumental in helping the patient to remain in a cherished home environment. Nurses feel that more staff and better resources would enable them to care for more such cases. Few recognise that heavier responsibilities of this kind would entail greater administrative control and closer monitoring of their work than that to which they are accustomed and is feasible under their present organisation.

The 'hospital at home' experiment in Peterborough demonstrated in broad terms the possibilities of increased and improved home care of the sick, through the appointment of a community nurse to manage the scheme. Such an appointment *could* not, however, carry with it guarantees to HAH patients of the levels and varieties of treatment and care they would have received had they been hospitalised. Nor *could* it ensure economic and optimum effective use of the scheme's personnel and resources. As a uniquely GP service, HAH Peterborough had primarily to be governed by demands made on it by individual GPs. Its nursing administration was broadly confined to matching available personnel with these demands, as far as possible according to nursing-assessed priorities.

Some district nurses in the locality of HAH Peterborough were disturbed by, and hostile to, the idea that hospital sector nurses might participate in the care of the scheme's patients (hostility of the kind sometimes shown to 'pain control' nurses, attached to some anti-cancer units which extend their services to patients at home). This reflects the extent to which some community nurses feel threatened by their organisationally stronger hospital colleagues. But, when we recall that district training is now mandatory for all domiciliary nurses, it is difficult to understand why there should be such strength of feeling against services aimed at enhancing home nursing skills. Indeed, had the Peterborough scheme achieved the identity of an integrated hospital/community service, a whole new field of possibilities in domiciliary nursing development might have been opened up.

Continuity of patient care is a notion now firmly grounded in some fields of medicine: for example, psychiatry and geriatric medicine. In many health districts, liaisive activities between hospital units and community nurses are highly effective; but in others poor co-ordination, breakdowns in communication and the absence of any single organisation holding overall responsibility for cases mean that patients and their families are often confused as to whether hospital or community nurses, or social workers, should be attending to particular needs.

Nowhere is the integrated approach to patient care more important than in the training and formation of the personnel who will spend most time with the patient. I have earlier discussed the role of patients' aides in HAH, describing the responsibilities of nurses in their training, formation and supervision – responsibilities which add important new dimensions to expectations of the nursing profession. These concern relationships between nurses, patients' aides and members of patients' entourages – family, friends, neighbours.

Even the most accomplished community nurse could not adequately fulfil all functions of patient care envisaged in 'hospital at home'. Apart from general and nursing administration, staff training and supervisory requirements (not to mention the daily care of the patient), the scheme is heavily committed to social casework – an ill defined and obscure skill, but one which, at minimum, requires wide and deep knowledge of welfare entitlements and understanding of social and psychosocial causes and consequences of illness.

Since health and social services reorganisation of the late 1960s and early 1970s many of the skills of medical social workers have been lost by health authorities. Their consequent increased reliance on health visitors for the performance of social work duties, once thought to be outside the latters' function, has not been accompanied by formal recognition of their new roles. It is to the credit of the health visiting profession that it has endeavoured to equip its members for these new responsibilities through more sensitive selection procedures and better training than previously applied.

Reorganisation, however, occurred at a time when health visitors and medical social workers were in the throes of training and role definition viz à viz each other. Taken together, the functions of both are far too wide and varied to be vested in one kind of worker alone. Those of health visitors in the field of health education, prevention and the early identification of persons at health risk, if carried out properly, are far too onerous for them to undertake at the same time casework and allied activities among the sick, inside and outside hospitals. There is still, therefore, a strong case for the selection and training of personnel of both distinct and different disciplines. This is discussed in more detail in the following chapter.

Relationships between district nurses and health visitors have always been uneasy. This is because they share the same training roots and have both originally practised as hospital nurses. Their respective roles in community nursing frequently overlap. More seriously, there are many occasions when neither district nurse nor health visitor feels that a particular task should be their respective responsibility.

The implications for nurses of a service which undertakes joint responsibility with patients' families for comprehensive home care, rather than one which provides only discrete items, are too fundamental to be skated over. Leaving aside implications for paramedical workers and overall health authority responsibility, the presence in patients' homes of multi-purpose aides under nursing management places on the nursing profession an obligation to resolve problems of conflicting expectations of its members, which hitherto it has left them to resolve for themselves as matters of individual conscience.

I have earlier described the duties of patients' aides as any which might be taken by a competent and caring member of the patient's family, were one available. Clearly such loose definition is open to all kinds of interpretation: by members of the family and others of the patient's entourage; by aides themselves and by the nurses supervising them. Under 'hospital at home' domiciliary care may involve working in all kinds of different home and social conditions, sometimes in the absence of modern conveniences, sometimes round the clock. It is thus crucial in the interests of both patients and those delegated responsibility for their care that conditions of employment and protection of the latter should be meticulously drawn up in full consultation with professional and trades' union representatives. No longer can the nursing profession, as sometimes occurs, disassociate itself from aspects of patients' care traditionally referred to as 'non-nursing'. I put it to readers, that all elements of patient care crucial to the most successful clinical management should be the co-ordinative responsibility of a nurse allocated charge of a case, a principle which at present applies among ward sisters in hospitals but not among community nurses. Of course, this applies only where members of the patient's family are not in a position, or do not wish, to play the co-ordinative role.

My claim that primary care teams are not appropriate bodies for the domiciliary care of patients suffering major disabling illness has to date met with hostility from some community nurses, although others have been among the first to recognise the fact. I hope that on reading these pages those hitherto hostile to the idea will agree that the setting up of secondary domiciliary care services for patients suffering major disabling illness is essential to their own greater contribution to the effective, humane care of their most needy patients.

References

(1) Bullough, V. L., and Bullough, B., *The Care of the Sick*, Croom Helm, London, 1979, p.57.
(2) Menzies, I. E. P., *A Case-study in the Functioning Social Systems as a Defence against Anxiety*, Tavistock Institute of Human Relations, London, undated.
(3) *Ibid.*, p. 118. See also Revans, R. W., 'The hospital as an organism: a study in communications and morale', paper presented at the 6th Annual International Meeting of the Institute of Management Sciences, September 1959.
(4) Menzies, *op. cit.*, p. 120.
(5) *Report of the Committee on Senior Nursing Staff Structure* (Chairman: B. Salmon), HMSO, London, 1966.
(6) Levitt, R., *The Reorganised National Health Service*, Croom Helm, London, 1976, pp. 126–43.
(7) *Report of the Committee on Local Authority and Allied Personal Social Services* (Chairman: F. Seebohm), Cmnd 3703, HMSO, London, 1968.
(8) *Report of the Working Party on Management Structures in the Local Authority Nursing Services* (Chairman: E. L. Mayston), HMSO, London, 1969.
(9) *Ibid.*

10 The other carers

Doctors alone hold clinical responsibility for their patients. It is up to them whether or not they concern themselves beyond the clinical field. The hospital patient does not necessarily suffer as a result of any failure to do so, because ward sisters are responsible for other aspects of care while the hospital machine provides for comprehensive resources which can be mobilised without as well as within medical prescription. It employs its own catering, domestic and portering staffs and paramedical workers; it organises social worker support; it draws upon the contributions of volunteers; and it lays down guidelines for the mobilisation of family support towards enhanced patient comfort.

Dependent patients at home, however, must rely on the perspicacity and energy of their GPs towards the identification of their non-clinical needs and the mobilisation of resources necessary to meet them when this task is beyond the capacity of the family. Only a minority of GPs meet these requirements satisfactorily. Most who attempt to do so rely largely on the efforts of their practice-attached nurses and health visitors towards this end.

Many essential aspects of patients' treatment and care, however, lie outside fields of both clinical medicine and nursing. This is recognised in hospitals, wherein paramedical and social work services have their own administrations; nurses may call upon, but do not themselves organise, volunteer services; and relatives and other members of the patients' own entourages have rights of direct access to general hospital administration. This does not and cannot occur under GP services because they are not covered by health authority administrations other than through community *nursing* divisions. Nevertheless, patients who are the concern of this book may well have requirements for paramedical, social worker and volunteer services equal to or higher than those of patients treated in hospitals. They certainly rely on the support of their families and friends to a greater extent.

To illustrate the complexity of making satisfactory home care arrangements for the dependent sick I have first chosen the case of Jane, a terminally ill patient.[1] In this case the family provided the principle support. Furthermore, they were articulate, well informed, and in a social position to themselves mobilise and co-ordinate the various services they were obliged to call upon in their attempts to avoid unwanted hospital admission. Nevertheless, the case demonstrates the need to incorporate into domiciliary patient provision facilities, including specialist facilities, additional to those available from GP and community nursing services.

Later in this book I shall refer to other cases, of kinds likely to be found on every average district nursing round, for which primary health care teams are neither properly organised nor equipped. Although all district nurses will be familiar with the kinds of cases I shall describe, it is unlikely, at a given time, that they would number many on a typical daily round, which is mostly concerned with the delivery of medically prescribed items which must take priority over time-consuming procedures.

Jane was 25 years old when it was found that cancer had spread to her bone marrow and her parents knew that death was imminent. Her illness had stretched over two years – a mixture of hope and hopes dashed by the discovery of further spread of the disease; operations; therapeutic treatments; pain; and brief spells when it seemed that, at least, the disease might be held in check.

Disastrous hospital experiences had threatened to sever Jane's bond with her parents which, despite her zest for independent living, had proved her mainstay of support in her bleakest moments. When she knew she was soon to die she was determined to enjoy the days left to her and to make her parents happy in the knowledge of her own happiness. They promised her that she should die at home with all the people and things around her which gave meaning to her life.

At home district nurses called several times daily, a health visitor every day. Her GP, who had known her since she was a child, promised to call at any time, night or day, if she wanted him. Jane was worried that she might be a burden on her parents, but she was reassured when she saw all the help they were receiving from the NHS. Friends came to visit her from all over the country.

Good as they were, the primary care workers in her area were not sufficiently experienced in pain control to be able to cope with Jane's case. It was she herself who finally suggested admission to a hospice where, she had read, few patients suffered and where the meaning of life was enriched in the face of death. It was fortunate in her case that hospice experience proved to be deeply enriching for both herself and her family. But such places are few and far between. In order to benefit from their facilities patient cases have to satisfy stringently applied criteria of admission (including short life expectation). Against their benefits must be measured the distress of separation from home and family, often at many miles distance, and the sacrifices which must be made by family and friends in order to be with the patient whenever they might be wanted. Without the presence of family and friends Jane's life would have lost its meaning. She was fortunate in being able to have them with her wherever she was. But had she been able to receive at home specialist services which are available in terminal care units towards relief and diversion from pain; had she felt confident that her presence at home did not place excessive strain on her parents, she might have died as she had wished – in her own home.

Ancillary workers

Many of us, with good reason, feel we owe debts of gratitude to health workers who are neither nurses nor doctors, but who, nevertheless, have contributed immeasurably to our relief and comfort in illness: ambulance drivers, with their calm competence and reassurance at the scene of an accident or other emergency; ward orderlies, porters and other ancillary personnel in hospitals, without whose backing doctors and nurses could not function properly.

'The ambulance journey was a nightmare, with every jolt, with every grimace, it was as if a knife was being driven into Jane, deeper every time. The younger man drove very slowly, very carefully. The older man stood up in the back with us, watching Jane's face, repeatedly telling the driver to go more gently . . . .'(2)

Patients at home are not currently provided with ancillary support by the NHS. Families are supposed to attend to needs of a non-nursing kind. Where need for such support is identified, it is (one hopes) arranged through LASSDs. Even in HAH Peterborough non-nursing personnel had to be employed as nursing auxiliaries – an arrangement which leaves ambiguous their commitment to duties categorically of a non-nursing kind.

Paramedical services

The need for improved domiciliary paramedical services throughout the NHS has been demonstrated in projects aimed at meeting the physiotherapy needs of house-bound patients.(3) These stress the importance of defining different organisational patterns required to provide for the needs of the disabled, chronically sick and handicapped, compared with those required to provide for the needs of the acutely ill. For the latter, the importance of involving hospital departments of physical medicine is emphasised: 'The focus in developing health services must be to provide the right treatment for the patient (assessment, advice, therapy and training) in the right place. This may sometimes be an institution and sometimes in the community, whether in the patient's home, health centre or elsewhere . . . '(4)

In many cases the 'right treatment' can be accurately determined only when all services involved can take part in determining an agreed programme. These services may include medical, paramedical, nursing and social work personnel, whom it is possible to call together inside hospitals at short notice, but this is virtually impossible outside.

Paramedical services have long been under-valued and under-used by the medical profession. (Many therapists of older generations will remember the difficulties of gaining footholds in their hospitals.) Only in the past decade or so have district therapy services been empowered by the DHSS but seldom staffed and equipped to provide adequate treatment for patients at home. As for the 'right treatment in the right place', it is sometimes questionable as to whether, on balance, some patients benefit at all from some hospital-centred treatments, their environmental conditions are so unsatisfactory. Many readers who have had cause to attend hospital for physiotherapy will remember long and uncomfortable journeys travelling to hospital by ambulance for a few minutes treatment, only to wait hours for the return journey, exposed to cold, draughts and other discomforts. Others will remember, perhaps, weeks spent in a hospital ward on traction, intended to repair an injured spine, suffering restless nights, mental tensions and anxieties, when, with modest support, similar treatment at home might have been more effective.

Domiciliary physiotherapy projects have been introduced to the NHS in recent years for a number of reasons: lack of open access by GPs to hospital-based physiotherapy services; transport difficulties; preference for home treatment by patients; advantages of instructing relatives in simple techniques of management and a treatment in home surroundings. One such project carried out in the Sheffield area between 1971 and 1974 pointed to advantages of mutually convenient times of treatment for patient and therapist, when, for example, the therapist does not have to rely on the department being open and a cubicle available; self-determined hours of work and flexible timetables – ideal for therapists with family commitments; and possibilities of case allocation within the therapist's home locality.[5]

Although some of these advantages apply to therapists rather than patients, the latter benefit in that paramedical skills are in short supply and must therefore be utilised as fully as possible.

The Sheffield project was held to have increased as a whole the efficiency of the primary health care teams in its area of operation. District nurses had already been engaged in simple physiotherapy procedures as part of their general duties. Now, with therapists to advise them, they could work more effectively themselves. But, despite its ackowledged success, the project was obliged to rely on charitable funding: the health authority responsible for it having been advised that it was not technically possible to make funds available for domiciliary physiotherapy.[6] Furthermore, as the Sheffield project progressed, it became evident that direct availability to GPs of paramedical services made health authority control over the latter extremely difficult.[7]

In some overseas services of the 'hospital at home' kind, paramedical workers, not nurses, function as case managers. For example, the Western Domiciliary Care (WDC) Service in South Australia was pioneered by the district hospital's department of physical medicine, whose medical director now also directs the WDC (see pages 62–3). In this case paramedical workers call for nursing aspects of care on the Royal District Nursing Society, which bases one of its nursing supervisors at WDC headquarters.

Experience of this service suggests that paramedical and social workers may, by and large, be more able than nurses in co-ordinating activities, the latter being more accustomed to working in isolation until problems of a non-nursing kind become too pressing to be ignored. Between them, paramedical and social workers have found it highly rewarding to their own roles to be able to develop support services comprising home helps, housekeepers, domiciliary helpers who have an elementary knowledge of home nursing, night attendants and sitters, 'handyman' help, and linen, appliance and meals provision; additionally, unsubsidised services such as hairdressing and gardening can be arranged through well wishers working for nominal charges and using volunteers who organise friendly visits and many other support activities. It seems to fit better with traditional expectations of nurses and with the aspirations of nurses themselves that they should have to concern themselves exclusively with aspects of patient care which they recognise to be of a professional nursing kind.

Whether 'hospital at home' and similar schemes are run by nurses or paramedical workers, the management of their patients' aides by members of one or the other group is essential. Where nurses occupy their management posts the services of these aides must be made available to paramedical and social workers, so that the latter can delegate to the aides, under their own instruction and supervision, simple tasks of a paramedical or social kind, and vice versa. In practice this has proved a highly effective way of conserving scarce skills of all professional disciplines, co-ordinating respective contributions in ways seldom apparent even in hospitals, where ancillary staffs are employed under different managements from those of professionals.

In HAH Peterborough paramedical workers found that they could instruct aides and members of the patient's family in certain procedures to be carried out at frequent and regular intervals which, had the patient had to attend hospital for them, would have been possible only two or three times a week. Occupational and speech therapists were able to assess the patient in a home environment soon after the onset of, for example, a stroke. They were convinced that in several cases this had resulted in earlier and more complete recovery than would have occurred had the patient been hospitalised.

Experiences of both the Sheffield project and HAH Peterborough confirm a need for consultant recommendation before paramedical services can be provided in the homes of patients. Apart from difficulties of health authority control over these services which would arise were independently contracted GPs able to prescribe them, many potentially disabling conditions require specialist investigation to ensure patient access to hospital-held rehabilitative material resources.

Social care of the home-bound sick

The presence of illness in the home places on families responsibilities they are spared when members are hospitalised. Many of these are of a social, not a medical or nursing, kind. Arguably, the social care of the sick, particularly those outside hospitals, is lower in level and quality now than prior to reorganisational changes, which removed from health authorities direct responsibility for the social care of sick persons.

Major organisational changes in personal social services provision took place in the early 1970s. After setting up local authority 'umbrella' social services departments (LASSDs) in line with the recommendations of the Seebohm Report, the Government of the time followed with clauses in its *NHS Reorganisation Act 1973* making obligatory the transfer of NHS medical and psychiatric social workers to these departments.[8] This represented a fundamental departure from previously held views that the social care of the sick was an integral part of health service responsibility.

Broadly, the move did not materially affect the extent of social worker support to hospitals. Some benefitted because they had not previously been able or willing to provide adequate social support services for patients in their care. Some lost out because they had been accustomed to higher levels of personnel and skills in their LASSDs than was now thought feasible or necessary. It did, however, ideologically reject concepts of specialist social workers integral to multi-disciplinary treatment teams. More seriously, it encouraged these teams to regard satisfaction of patients' social needs as being outside their own responsibilities.

Pressure from hospital doctors for the retention of social workers (now employed by local authorities) was largely due to medical and administrative concern about the blocking of beds by long-stay patients. However differently individual doctors and hospital social workers themselves might have hitherto evaluated the work of the latter, facilitating difficult discharges is and always has been generally considered by hospital professionals and administrators to be their most useful function.

In the main, GPs have never regarded social work as an essential element of their practices. Their responsibilities to their patients are purely of a clinical kind. District nurses and health visitors are usually at hand to relieve them of non-medical worries. Furthermore, LASSDs are supposed to deal with social aspects of need. Moreover, GPs do not have to concern themselves with patients who are blocking hospital beds. Indeed, they would have far more problems on their hands if many such patients were discharged. The fact that blocked beds create problems in gaining admissions is, by and large, a less immediate consideration.

Historically, social worker aspirations to break away from medical domination were satisfied when health and welfare departments headed by medical officers of health were abolished under the NHS Reorganisation Act of 1973 to make way for organisationally separate local government environmental health, community health and personal social services departments. Environmental health includes the removal of refuse, sanitary inspection of public hygiene, orders under the *Clean Air Act 1958*, open spaces, public baths, disinfestation, inspections under the *Food and Drugs Act 1955* and under the *Offices Shops and Railway Premises Act 1963*. Community health care (excluding that particular to GP services under Family Practitioner Committees) is, following the requirements of the *Local Government Act 1972* (Section 112), the responsibility of district community physicians employed by health authorities of central, not local, government. Personal social services are defined according to local government statute which, by definition, does not deal with matters of physical or mental illness.

Three-way organisational rupture of services at one time embodied in the functions of local authority health and welfare departments, may have been successful in breaking up monolithic institutions which stunted the growth of personal social services in favour of those of an environmental health and medical kind. But, in themselves now becoming monolithic institutions, embracing wide and often disparate statutory functions, social services' departments now inhibit the development of integrated health/social services according to specialist requirements: for example, for the deaf, blind, mentally and/or physically handicapped, children at risk and, the subjects of this book, persons suffering major, incapacitating illness.[10]

Only the last-mentioned essentially require organisational provision based on medical treatment services, although illness in a member of any of the other groups may change the nature of service required, from non-medical to one embodying medical treatment. Since no local authority is now empowered to provide the latter it follows that health authorities should be obliged to ensure satisfaction of all patients minimum essential social needs. They are not. Only in hospitals does this obligation stand.

The *NHS Reorganisation Act 1973* anticipated the continuing need for social services support to the health service through its Clauses 12(2) and 18(4)(a). Clause 12(2) placed a vague responsibility on health authorities to decide how much social worker support they wanted and on local authorities to determine how much they considered reasonable and were able to provide. Clause 18(4)(a) defined social workers as persons appointed to carry out statutory functions under the Social Services Act of 1970. Taken together, these two clauses effectively put an end to medical social work as an integral part of patient treatment and care. More seriously, it effectively absolved health authorities from any statutory responsibility for basic and special social support for the sick outside hospitals, even where this might be crucial to successful treatment and nursing care.

In undertaking to provide parallel alternatives to general hospital admission for certain patients, HAH Peterborough was brought face to face with problems of divided health and social services. It had the task of integrating into multi-disciplinary patterns of care elements which, following 1974 reorganisation, were now the responsibility of LASSDs, not health authorities.[11] It found solutions to some of these problems, for example, commode-emptying, by employing patients' aides under nursing management. But still there remained those of, for example, the handling of patients' monies and other private affairs. Matters of this kind expressly outside the functions of nurses should be the concern of qualified social workers when patients or their families are not in positions to handle them. Although not featured in research findings on HAH Peterborough, it is likely that lack of social work provision integral to the scheme influenced the extent to which patients with social, in addition to medical, problems could be accepted by it.

Financial support for the home-bound sick

Patients in NHS hospitals, we recall, are looked after free of charge whilst undergoing treatment. Since 'hospital at home' seeks to provide a parallel to in-patient care, and since there is currently no NHS obligation to meet the non-nursing needs of the home-bound, the most important social work function in HAH Peterborough was to ensure that its patients received material and financial support to which they might be entitled, or eligible for, from statutory and voluntary sources outside the NHS: for example, extra heating allowances; nourishment grants; linen, clothing and other material supplements and replacements; aids to daily living – all enhance numbers of patients and their families who, given the chance, would exercise options in favour of home, rather than hospital, treatment.

Outside the statutory sector a wealth of possibilities exists whereby patients might be enabled to opt for home care alternatives otherwise denied to them. Charitable and non-profit-making organisations of many varieties are standing by ready to relieve families of some of the burden of illness in the home, if only those in need of their help might be identified. A major failure of the NHS is its organisational inability to make optimum use of ready and willing contributions from the voluntary sector. This applies particularly outside hospitals.

Despite its social work shortcomings, HAH Peterborough managed to demonstrate one important way in which financial help, traditionally available only to hospital patients, might be made available to patients at home. This is of particular historical interest to students of British health care, because it relates to times when many working people relied on member-ship of provident societies for financial cover at times of illness. It also demonstrates how hospital admission has, over the years, attracted financial benefits more favourable to the patient than has provision for their home care.

The Hospital Savings Association (HSA) was one of the few provident societies to survive the creation of the NHS, drawing together thousands of small hospital-centred organisations into a centralised service, operating a vast network of local groups preserving a spirit of independence and self-reliance. As the HSA is tied to the hospital movement, there is financial inducement for HSA members to be hospitalised in preference to home care. Recognising that this factor might weigh heavily with HSA members in Peterborough who might have preferred hospital to HAH for this reason, the HSA agreed to pay benefits during a stay in HAH at the same rates as that payable had members been admitted to hospital. The arrangement held for the duration of the three-year project only on condition that members were offered genuine options between general hospital admission and HAH.[12] This major concession on the part of the HSA was a measure of its appreciation of the status of HAH.

Volunteers

Despite adequate treatment, personal care, domestic help and financial security, many home-bound patients live lives of loneliness, bereft of the extra comforts which supportive families and/or hospitals usually provide. An important role for HAH social workers lies in the organisation of voluntary and neighbourly help, so that it can be called upon at immediate notice should the need arise. Wide varieties of voluntary organisations in many localities will readily help the sick outside their memberships provided that professionals will accept responsibility for the arrangements. Some will help patients suffering particular medical conditions only: for example, multiple sclerosis; rheumatism; arthritis; diabetes; chest and heart diseases. Their special value lies in members' first-hand experiences of the particular condition. Other groups – for example, the Women's Royal Voluntary Services; the Red Cross and the Order of St John; Age Concern; the Council for the Disabled; Rotary Clubs – will provide help regardless of the nature of illness, as long as other circumstances of the case merit it. Still others – for example, church and neighbourhood associations; mothers' unions; townswomen's guilds; senior citizens' clubs – will appeal among their members for offers of help for patients who are lonely or otherwise lacking in comfort, although their primary functions do not extend outside their own memberships.

It is customary for social workers to apply direct on behalf of their clients to these various organisations when a particular case of hardship arises, or else through multi-purpose volunteer bureaux which keep lists of volunteers. Both practices tend to produce patchy, sometimes unreliable, response, not always sensitive to the particular stresses of major illness. Home-bound patients suffering the latter without adequate support from their families may need voluntary help *co-ordinated* with that provided by the responsible statutory body covering the patient's treatment needs.

The potential need for voluntary help among the homebound sick is wide and varied. Examples include sitting with the patient when family members, neighbours or friends, cannot be present; reading, and providing other diversions; changing library books; transporting frail, incapacitated loved ones to visit patients; hedge-cutting (perhaps the view from the sickroom window is blocked) and other gardening; care of pets; comforting the bereaved.

Perhaps more important, even, than the contributions of

volunteers whilst patients remain the responsibilities of HAH are their potential to develop more lasting relationships when patients ultimately leave its protection. Through these, further breakdown in health among the lonely and isolated can be avoided, whilst daily lives may be enriched by new friendships and widened social horizons.

The functions of HAH social workers in the enlistment, training and mobilisation of volunteers to work among the home-bound sick are therefore of a specialised kind. But, we recall, at present there is no provision for their specialised training for the task: while the only existing organisational setting which lends itself to specialised practice is in hospitals.

Voluntary work among patients suffering major and terminal illness is fraught with dangers from the selection and training of volunteers onward. Close investigation into motives and backgrounds is necessary, but, at the same time, this can be destructive to warm informal relationships. Volunteer and patient must be happily matched case for case. Many volunteers resent too close a rein on their activities. Yet, they like to feel that professional help is readily at hand if they are in difficulties. Too often the careless and insensitive use of volunteers results in loss of their services. Since volunteers in HAH are likely to come into close daily contact with nurses and patients' aides, the social workers responsible for their mobilisation and monitoring have the dual responsibility of ensuring smooth relationships between them and HAH personnel, as well as patients and their families.

Conclusion

On reading this chapter one might well question the potential effect on the patient of seemingly limitless numbers and varieties of persons – doctors, nurses, paramedical and social workers, patients' aides, volunteers – converging on the patient's household. Recognising the dangers, 'hospital at home' schemes must plan their work so that the minimum number of necessary visiting personnel are involved in each case. The idea being that nurse and patient's aide should provide the mainstay of support not forthcoming from the family; nurses, paramedical and social workers as far as possible utilise patients' aides where their own professional presence is not essential for treatment reasons. Visits from volunteers should of course only be at the wishes of patient and family. Given these conditions, the greater the availability, in numbers and varieties, of personnel potentially available to participate in patient care, the greater the prospects of providing care of a kind likely to hasten recovery and/or provide relief from pain and other distress.

References and notes

(1) Zorza, R., and Zorza, V., *A Way to Die: Living to the End*, André Deutsch, London, 1980.
(2) *Ibid.*
(3) Waters, W. H. R., *et al.*, 'Organising a physiotherapy service in general practice', *Journal of the Royal College of General Practitioners*, 1975, **25**, 576–584.
(4) *Ibid.*
(5) *Ibid.*
(6) *Ibid.*
(7) *Ibid.*
(8) *Report of the Committee on Local Authority Allied Personal Social Services* (Chairman: F. Seebohm), Cmnd 3703, HMSO, London, 1968; 'Social work support for the health service', DHSS Circular LASSL (73), 47; *Social Work Support for the Health Service*, HMSO, London, 1974; *The National Health Service Reorganisation Act 1973*, HMSO, London, 1973.
(9) *NHS Reorganisation Act 1973, op. cit.*
(10) *Ibid.*, Section (8) (i).
(11) *Ibid.*, Section (8) (v), Clauses 12(2) and 18(4)(a). NB: The author was a founder member and chairperson of the Health Service Social Workers Group from 1971 to 1974. She holds records of the Group's activities at that time, including counsel's opinion that Clause 18(4)(a) of the NHS Reorganisation Bill was invalid. The Group felt unable to pursue this through the Courts because the terms of Clause 12(2) abolished health authorities' rights to employ their own social workers.
(12) Minutes of the meeting of the Steering Group for the Peterborough Hospital at Home three-year pilot scheme, 25 October 1978, Item 32: Progress Report.

11 How to get your local 'hospital at home' service

Some readers may feel that, by and large, existing arrangements for home care in Britain have served us well so 'why make changes'?

Only when we have personally experienced major illness in the home, in the absence of kinds and levels of help we felt were needed but could not obtain, are we likely to have strong feelings that changes are necessary.

As for hospital admission, while, in the past, we may have been able to persuade ourselves that the doctor would not have recommended it had it not been necessary, we now have to remind ourselves more and more that there are occasions when doctors *cannot* know what is for the best in our particular cases: that, ultimately, the responsibility for decision making rests with the patient.

Opportunities for this decision making are far from realistic. Agreed, home environments have important advantages over those of hospitals. But, whilst at home and exclusively the clinical responsibilities of our GPs, we forfeit rights of access to many of the resources (hospital-held) potentially able to help in our recoveries. Only if health authority responsibility were extended to GP services could we exercise these rights of access without opting for hospital admission.

It would be reassuring to know that, should we become ill and our families unable to look after us, others representing our interests would come forward to make sure that, as far as possible, arrangements for our care met with our own aspirations. This seldom occurs. If families are not of kinds, and in positions, to act as patients' watchdogs, the latter usually have to fit in with what the system decides is best for them.

Nevertheless, we do have watchdogs in the NHS. Additionally, diverse outside organisations exist to protect the interests of various groups of disadvantaged persons, including those in which illness prevails. Unfortunately, the extent to which NHS watchdogs and these organisations are able to take concerted action in favour of improved health care for the population as a whole is extremely limited.

Community health councils (CHCs) exist to represent consumer interests in the NHS. They are (or should be) set up in every health authority district, and operate with varying degrees of drive and competence. Some are highly effective in the work they do, but their scope is restricted: partly by limitations on powers invested in them; partly by the fact that pressures on them from the establishment side, even if not reinforced by these limitations, make it difficult for them to be ethically exact in their roles as watchdogs of consumer interests. Added to this, in their peripheral activities on the borders between carers and cared-for, members of CHCs inevitably have divided sympathies between the two sides. Furthermore, few of their members have knowledge of NHS origins, structure, organisation and mode of operation sufficient to give them the confidence necessary to pursue enquiry reaching the roots of many problems and to search out lasting solutions to these problems. Most significant of all perhaps, in restrictions to CHCs' effectiveness, is the fact that they have no rights of enquiry into GP services. Effectively, this means that they are virtually powerless to work towards improved treatment services outside hospitals.

Even so, CHCs do possess powers of influence over potentially all aspects of NHS activity, inside and outside hospitals, which few appear to use. They can enlist support from their MPs; use the press and other media to articulate their views; and work through their national body, which has powers to take up matters of widespread concern with the DHSS and the Government.[1] It is, therefore, to CHCs that 'hospital at home' must look, both for understanding of its concepts, aims and possibilities and, ultimately, for public understanding of HAH and its potential in providing parallel alternatives to general hospital admission.

Outside the NHS many organisations set up to protect and pursue the interests of various groups of disadvantaged persons have proud records of vigorous and enterprising campaigning, not only on behalf of individuals, but also towards the universal good of those whom they claim to represent. For proof of this, one only has to study the histories, for example, of organisations set up to help the terminally ill, the elderly, the mentally and/or physically handicapped, the blind, the deaf, and sick children. Although, other than in the case of the terminally ill, they do not insist on strict definitions of illness before intervening in a case, they are all particularly concerned about what happens to those whom they set out to help when illness is present. However, the diversity of patients, in terms of age and medical conditions, and taking into account other residual disabilities, makes it difficult or impossible for discrete organisations to enter into concerted dialogue with medical treatment services organised largely according to medical specialisms.

Between them the various organisations mentioned above and CHCs could do much to persuade Government and the DHSS of the need to introduce to the NHS a secondary home care service parallel to general hospital admission. But, since the NHS is bound to look to possible economic and other establishment-favouring aspects of any proposed innovation, rather than those primarily of patient interest, representatives of patients themselves need to be impeccably equipped with the facts of their case before putting it before official bodies. They also need to be crystal clear about the respective requirements of patients who (or whose families) are able to co-ordinate the various elements of treatment care and basic support they need, and those who must rely on statutory help toward this.

However well researched and effective in presentation, any campaign in favour of tighter health authority control over community sectors activity than at present is certain to meet with resistance from professionals jealous of their individual freedoms. CHCs and other patient interest bodies motivated towards the provision of domiciliary patient services involving increased resource allocations outside hospitals (and, therefore, increased health authority control over the regulation of these resources) would be well advised to understand both the true extent of resistance and the extent of professional support to be antici-pated, in the event of a campaign in favour of enhanced domiciliary provision for the sick.

Although the lay public may be under the impression that any departure from concepts of independent GP practice under the NHS would meet with insurmountable resistance from the medical profession, this is by no means necessarily the case. Doubtless most GPs of the older generations with well established, thriving practices would object to changes. But, as I have pointed out in chapter 8, a large percentage of GPs of the younger generations and emerging doctors seeking their first permanent appointments would willingly accept monitoring and control (outside uniquely clinical matters) from health authorities, given better access to health facilities for their patients than are currently available to GPs independently contracted to FPCs. Given access to general hospital beds, which might well be anticipated in the event of their health authority employment, the percentage would undoubtedly rise.

Hospital specialists, already accountable to health authorities, are seemingly satisfied with their salaried appointments under health authorities, so their potential involvement in HAH presents no organisational problem. But, since many currently rely in part on domiciliary visiting for their private practices, some objections to extensions of their health authority commitments in the domiciliary field might be anticipated. Furthermore, some might question the extent to which their involvement with domiciliary services could be justified in terms of time and economy. (Arguably, it is cheaper and quicker to treat patients *en masse* than under separate roofs.) However, HAH envisages that most of its cases would be susceptible to outpatient attendance for most specialist interventions: and the fact that the scheme would relieve many hospital beds of patients not essentially requiring them, leaving them free for others who did, must be weighed against that of possibly uneconomic domiciliary visits.

Both specialists and GPs would wish to be clear about mutual relationships under HAH, since, under current NHS arrangements, specialists participate in patients' treatments outside hospitals only at the invitation of the GP in the case, an arrangement which lacks any formal organisational backing.

Some district nurses would object to HAH on the grounds that it would limit varieties of cases traditionally included in their daily rounds, and that it might interfere with the nature of nurse–GP practice attachments. Some would resist the idea of closer management control and monitoring of their work than currently applies.

Despite the fact that district nursing qualifications are now mandatory for personnel working in the homes of patients (and this would apply to HAH nurses), some district nurses faced with HAH proposals appear unable to visualise hospital-based home care arrangements which do not rely on hospital-based nurses lacking such qualifications. Only those of us intimately acquainted with traditional relationships between hospital and community nurses will fully appreciate the extent to which the latter guard their territories from incursion by the former.

Experience so far suggests that hospital nurses would welcome the introduction of HAH to the NHS. Aware of restrictions on their effectiveness in institutional settings, many would be prepared to undertake the district training necessary for their participation in HAH activities. Others, preferring more technically demanding hospital positions (for example, in operating theatres and intensive care units and as ward sisters) would welcome HAH as a means of freeing hospital beds for more clinically satisfying cases than is presently feasible.

Politicians and administrators may feel uneasy about HAH proposals because they know from past experience how notoriously difficult it is to keep control over amenities freely accessible to GPs. They may gain reassurance from close study of means by which French hospital administrations and financing mechanisms keep control over *hospitalisation à domicile* (see chapter 5).

As most CHC members will be aware, many innovations have been introduced to community sectors of the NHS in recent years, in efforts both to economise on hospital beds and to add to the benefits of home care for the patient. They have led to deeper awareness and understanding of problems of home care than has ever before been apparent in official NHS thinking. Through their experience of problems of *ad hoc* piecemeal primary care arrangements, those responsible for such innovations have much to offer proponents of the more structured approaches to home care suggested in this book. This experience, added to that of CHCs and other consumer interest organisations deeply aware of public suspicion of innovations aimed at avoiding unwanted hospital admissions (unwanted by patient or by hospital personnel?) could help lay permanent foundations for the establishment of secondary domiciliary care schemes capable of satisfying both professional and lay aspirations towards the avoidance of unwanted hospital admissions.

In chapter 7 I demonstrated attempts at continuing care between hospital and community health services through examples including MacMillan Continuing Care Services (CCSs) sponsored jointly by the National Society for Cancer Relief (NSCR) and the health authorities in whose districts they have been set up (see pages 108–9). To recapitulate: it is not the function of these services to 'take over' patient cases from GPs and community nurses, but, rather, to act as catalysts, providing, (subject to the agreement of GP and nurse), medical, nursing, social and/or volunteer input, according to the particular requirements of each CCS case.

The surge of growth in MacMillan CCSs during the past decade has been dramatic. Geographically, they now cover half the UK.[2] But the percentage of all terminally ill cancer sufferers in the UK aspiring to home care and provided with it through these units is extremely low. There are four main reasons for this:

(1) General hospital specialists are often reluctant to make referrals to them, feeling they have a moral duty to keep their patients in their own units through the terminal stages of illness.

(2) CCSs are highly selective of the cases they accept. If an estimated life expectation is of more than say, six months, they may refuse a case as being a premature referral. If it is very short they may refuse it on the grounds that it would be unfair to subject a patient to the inevitable stresses of removal from one hospital unit to another. (The home care element, which is the main appeal of CCSs for some patients, usually follows rather than precedes case assessment at a CCS centre.)

(3) For home care to be realistic in a CCS case, the patient needs to live in fairly close proximity to the centre, otherwise staff cannot keep the case under close and frequent supervision.

(4) Many terminally ill patients prefer as far as possible to live their lives out in an accustomed environment rather than seek a strange one.

Undoubtedly, many terminally ill patients are well provided for by CCSs plus community nursing and social services of the *ad hoc* kind. This is usually because they have strong and articulate family support, whereby a member of the family acts as co-ordinator of the various services involved. But, as CCS personnel would be among the first to agree, there are many cases in which patients have no alternative but to remain resident in CCSs because family contributions plus those of primary care cannot provide the care and support requisite to their particular needs.

I therefore put it to CHCs and other patient interest groups that, despite their advantages, MacMillan and similar CCSs, selective of their cases according to diagnositc considerations, are intrinsically incapable of making optimal provision for the group of patients they seek to help. In order to do so they would require access, in every health district, to a general domiciliary care service like HAH, able to assume responsibility for cases where higher levels and wider varieties of support than can be provided by primary health care services are required.

GPs and community nurses will need no introduction to the kinds of cases for which primary care services are improperly organised to cope adequately. Hospital doctors and nurses will already be well aware of those where the patient is resistant to hospital disciplines and where there is no prime treatment reason for admission. But, since a health system founded on centuries of tradition and orientated in favour of hospitals is unlikely to produce from within pressures sufficient to redress the balance in favour of more and better home care for the sick, it is to the lay public and their health representatives that we must look for leadership in campaigning towards this.

Since lay readers may not be clear as to the varieties of cases potentially resistant to hospital admission but not susceptible to primary care responsibility, I have exampled below a cross-section of my own aquaintance.

The particular cases I mention were among 30 referred to HAH Peterborough in its first six months of operation, from November 1978 to April 1979. All these cases would have had to be hospitalised had it not been for the presence of HAH, despite the fact that Peterborough community nursing services rate high compared, perhaps, with most others throughout the NHS. I have, of course, used fictitious names and, where necessary, made minor changes in case histories to avoid possibilities of case identification:

Miss Posy Green was a bizarre, exasperating, character who taxed the patience and ingenuity of HAH Peterborough staff. She had on numerous occasions been admitted to psychiatric hospitals, usually with disastrous consequences. On the last occasion she had set fire to the ward curtains. A month previous to her referral to HAH she had fallen on the ice, fracturing her wrist. Since then her plaster had been replaced three times, because she persisted in getting it wet. Now her arm was sore and in danger of infection. Miss Green adamantly refused hospital admission. In any case, the district hospital was not keen on admitting her.

Two weeks with Miss Green's case strained nurses and patients' aides almost beyond endurance. But at least they managed to keep her plaster dry until the fracture was mended.

Mr Osborne was already under treatment from his GP when he had a stroke. From past experience the GP knew he would not agree to hospital admission. At the same time, his wife would not be able to cope with him and his case would have been too demanding for the practice-attached nurse's attentions. Rapid but thorough assessment by HAH nurse and social worker suggested need for a concentration of paramedical services from early on in Mr Osborne's admission to the scheme. Some persuasion was needed to convince his GP to prescribe this so soon after onset of the stroke. He had been accustomed to considering rehabilitation only after initial treatment had been completed. In the event, the patient's multi-disciplinary care from the time of admission on brought about his immediate and rapid improvement. Doctor and therapists remarked that this could never have been achieved in a hospital environment.

As the weeks wore on Mr Osborne's daughter became anxious about the strain on her mother of looking after her father at home. She remarked that he had always used her mother as a 'doormat' and was now beginning to take advantage of being treated as an invalid. Hoping to give Mrs Osborne a break, and, at the same time, to complete the process of rehabilitation, the GP approached the hospital geriatrician for a place in his day hospital. Unfortunately, there was at the time industrial action among the ambulance drivers of the area, making a daily journey impossible. Anxious to be helpful, the geriatrician therefore agreed to admit him, with the intention of arranging his attendance at the day hospital from the ward. In the event this proved disastrous. Within four days Mr Osborne became incontinent, refused to eat or speak, and literally turned his face to the wall. His family begged for his return back to the care of HAH, following which he rapidly recovered again. Now, however, he was far less demanding of his wife. Two weeks later, only two months after the onset of his stroke, he was able to walk unattended, with his walking frame, round the garden, inspecting the early crocuses and making plans for the spring planting.

Mr Fowler, in his late 70s, had never previously been seriously ill, when, shovelling his way out of a snowdrift, he suffered a cerebrovascular accident. Now wholly paralysed, he was unable to discuss the possibility of hospital admission. But, his wife said, he would never willingly have called a doctor, let alone entered hospital. Anyway, his GP felt he was too ill to be moved, especially in view of the weather conditions at the time. So he asked HAH if it could accept his case.

The case presented major problems for both HAH nurse and social worker. The former was faced with the problem of organising round the clock care, while the latter, within a space of hours, had to obtain financial and material help towards coverting a primitive, ill equipped, one-bedroomed cottage to provide not only for Mr Fowler, but also privacy and comfort for his wife, an invalid herself, and facilities for the patients' aides and various members of the patient's family who had agreed to participate in his care.

A corner of the family living-room was converted into a sick bay. From there Mr Fowler, now failing fast but responsive and clearly appreciative of the attention he was receiving, enjoyed the comfort of familiar surroundings and faces until his death two weeks after his admission to HAH.

George Saunders, a bachelor in his 50s, had been off work only a few weeks when he was told by his doctor that tests had revealed an inoperable lung cancer. He took the news philosophically, but refused hospital saying he would rather die at home. He lived alone and his nearest relatives lived some miles away. But his neighhours, a couple with two young children, said they would do all they could to help, provided HAH would take responsibility for his case. Between them, a niece, neighbours, patient's aide and nurse were on hand night and day, nevertheless respecting his wish to be left on his own as far as was possible.

As had been expected, Mr Saunder's condition deteriorated rapidly. Twelve days after his admission to HAH he died in the middle of the night.

This case revealed a shocking lack of suitable provision for medical attention to seriously ill, home-bound patients during unsocial hours. Despite the determination of HAH Peterborough to ensure that all its patients should receive requisite medical attention, day and night, it proved impossible to persuade local GPs to commit themselves to more than their traditional arrangements for domiciliary visiting. In Mr Saunder's case, the GP was off duty when the patient's condition suddenly deteriorated late one evening. The HAH nurse's call for medical assistance was referred to a deputising service. When the deputising doctor finally arrived on the scene, several hours after the call went out, the patient was already dead. In any event he had no previous knowledge of the case and made no effort to examine the deceased man physically, console relatives or help in any other way. He left the house within ten minutes of calling, saying he would arrange for completion of the death certificate in the morning. What, we asked ourselves, would have happened had HAH not been present on the case?

The GP was of the opinion of that Mr Watson, an obese man in his 80s, was 'putting on' his many symptoms of ill health. But when HAH Peterborough was called in the problem was real enough. The previous night the patient had fallen down the narrow flight of stairs in his cottage. Unable to get help, his wife had had to leave him, wedged at the bottom, all night. Cold and shocked, he had with considerable difficulty been dragged back up the stairs. He was now lying in bed, doubly incontinent, apathetic and apparently unaware of his surroundings.

Mr Watson's wife, a lively lady in her early 70s, enjoyed a busy social life at local clubs and bingo hall. She clearly resented being tied to the house to look after her husband. She was angry that the GP had not attempted to get him into hospital (in any case he would not have agreed to this) and was now unco-operative and resentful at the idea of HAH intervention. Strictly speaking HAH should not have accepted this case since Mrs Watson was not happy at the idea of home care for her husband. But, at the time of its referral, we had not been able to gain agreement from all local GPs participating in our experiment that family attitudes as well as clinical considerations would ultimately determine patients' environments of treatment. While some GPs in the locality readily accepted the need for clear identification of family wishes, others insisted that it went without saying that arrangements they made for their patients would take these into account.

Mr Watson died a couple of weeks after his fall. Family and neighbours were so impressed by the help received from HAH that they clubbed together to make a generous donation towards the setting up of a 'Samaritan fund' for HAH Peterborough, to be used for extra comforts for patients in special need.

Mr and Mrs Baxter, both in their 70s, suffered mental illness, she only intermittently, he from senile dementia. By and large she coped well with her husband's occasionally violent behaviour. But now, with a broken arm, she found it impossible.

HAH allocated a patient's aide to the case twice a day, four hours in all, supervised by a nurse who made brief visits twice daily. In this way the scheme was able to avert a hospital admission, which would probably have been catastrophic for both patients: for him, because on previous occasions his admission had exacerbated his condition; for her, because on other occasions he had suffered bouts of uncontrollable violence vented on his wife for several weeks following his discharge.

John, in his late 20s, had some years earlier sustained grave injuries as a result of which he was paralysed from the neck down. He needed little in the way of treatment, but his nursing care included skilled procedures, including, for example, manual faecal evacuation. From time to time he was subject to unpredictable collapse requiring urgent medical intervention.

John was lovingly cared for by devoted parents. On previous occasions when they needed a break he had been admitted to hospital. This he detested. So when HAH came on the scene it seemed the ideal solution for his care whilst his parents spent a month abroad with relatives.

This case caused some controversy among steering group members of the Peterborough experiment. Some held that, since his hospital admission was not justified for medical reasons, a case

could not be made for offering John an option between hospital
and HAH care. But reason prevailed on the grounds that, had
HAH facilities *not* been available, John would have had to be
admitted to the district hospital.

Another feature special to John's case was the fact that, over
the years, he had been regularly visited by the same district
nurses of the primary care team in his locality. Knowing him so
well, they enjoyed his confidence and friendship and had learned
the best ways of helping him to cope with his problems.
Flexibility of HAH operation enabled these nurses to continue in
the case, whilst HAH itself provided the patients' aide support
and overall case co-ordination necessary to ensure that someone
would always be present to fill gaps in his attendance caused by
his parents' absence.

Mrs Jones, aged 40 years, had recently undergone surgery,
radiotherapy and chemotherapy at the regional cancer unit some
50 miles from her home. The doctors now pronounced her
condition untreatable and took the view that she might have no
more than a month or so to live. Her husband, mother-in-law and
two grown up daughters living away from home between them
kept the home going, looked after Mrs Jones, lately confined to
her bed, and her 7 year old daughter. It now looked as if either
Mrs Jones, Snr might lose her part-time job, upon which, as a
widow, she was financially dependent, or the patient might have
to enter hospital, an idea distressing to her and her family. In
accepting responsibility for her case, HAH hoped to enable her to
spend her remaining days at home and among her family.

The scheme provided her with an adjustable bed erected in a
corner of the living-room. In the presence of HAH she pulled out
of her depression of the past month, spent isolated in an upstairs
bedroom. Her husband was now able to get his sleep on those
nights he was not 'on duty', knowing that someone else was
present to attend to her needs. Her mother-in-law, now only one
of a rota of carers, was able to resume her part-time job.

As her spirits rose, Mrs Jones gained in health. She began to
take an interest in her appearance, wearing for the first time the
wig supplied to conceal loss of hair, a side-effect of chemotherapy.
She watched TV with the family, joined in her daughter's games
and other activities, and learned to walk again. She and the

patients' aide in the case became firm friends; neighbours rallied round. It was a memorable day for her when her wish to attend a family wedding came true. In the event, she survived almost a year of happiness shared with her family, in the knowledge that her presence at home created none of the problems she had thought would stem from her resistance to hospital admission.

A variety of diagnoses have been included in the above examples, ranging from broken bones plus mental disturbance, through strokes, to those of terminal cancer. Durations of patient stay in the cases described ranged from a week to two months, but would have been extended for as long as the patient required continuing care of the HAH type. Three of the eight patients whose cases are described above died whilst in the Peterborough scheme – a measure of its need to parallel general hospital services.

There could have been no greater testimony to the need in Britain for services like HAH than the esteem the Peterborough experiment won from its patients and their families. It was this esteem which gained it so much lay support in the area: support which led to health authority agreement to make it a permanent part of its amenities (albeit one which ultimately lost its identity as a *bona fide* general hospital alternative because local GPs would not accept the administrative measures necessary to enable the AHA to keep control of resources it would have had to allocate outside its hospital sector in order that this might be achieved).

Whether or not certain patients in the UK are ultimately provided with parallel alternatives to institutional care through the existence in every locality of units of the kind described by this book could be largely determined by CHCs. Through these councils the many other organisations who watch the interests of the sick could exert pressures on politicians, professionals and administrators, often resistant to lay participation in health matters, towards domiciliary patient provision avoiding the need for unwanted and unnecessary hospitalisations.

One thing is clear. If fit and active members of the public do not act positively to further and protect the interests of patients too ill to act for themselves, professional interests not always fully cognisant of patients needs will prevail.

References

(1) Levitt, R., *The Reorganised National Health Service*, Croom Helm, London, 1976, pp. 190–5.
(2) *Cancer Relief News*, Spring and Summer 1983.

12 Summary, conclusions and prospects for the future

My studies on 'hospital at home' have led me to conclude need for radical NHS reorganisation before reforms can be introduced which could offer consumers optimum benefits from nationalised health care. This reorganisation would have to cover arrangements for the prevention of illness as well as for its cure.

I have found that existing services organised, respectively, within hospital and community health authority divisions, with GP services organisationally outside both, fail to recognise radical differences between arrangements necessary for optimal illness prevention and optimal treatment and care of the sick.

Prevention is a responsibility shared with statutory organisations other than those of a predominantly medical kind: for example, social, educational, employment and housing organisations. The NHS, uniquely concerned with the prevention and cure of illness, requires structure and organisation enabling it to respond humanely, quickly and effectively, both to needs connected with the health of the nation as a whole and to those of individuals suffering from or vulnerable to illness in particular.

The NHS has now been in existence long enough for us to reach conclusions as to its effectiveness to date in both directions, compared with that of other health systems – some of which claim success equal to or greater than our own, through integrated treatment services spanning boundaries between hospital and community, whilst developing preventive services largely independently of those of treatment.

In its early days the NHS offered prospects of health care which, it was justly held, could not be matched by any other health system of Western or Western-style democracies. It demonstrated the many advantages which universal treatment

and care, free at the time of delivery, could offer over systems
requiring financial enquiry and/or means testing before entitlement to services could be established. It has been the source of
inspiration for many innovations in the statutory provisions of
countries less advanced than Britian in matters of health and
welfare. Yet it is now under threat of erosion, even dismantle-
ment. Nationwide economic recession is a commonly held reason
for this. But deeper analysis suggests that there may also be more
fundamental reasons why the NHS is failing to live up to its
original promise. Does the NHS in its present form have the
structure, organisation and capacity to ensure that its resources
are used to best possible effect? If it is to survive it will have to
produce evidence of economic, effective and humane operation,
equal to or greater than that of the most advanced of other health
systems.

Research on 'hospital at home' has led me to conclude that
there exist four major features preventing optimum NHS
operation: (1) basic reliance on independently contracted GPs,
over whose services health authorities have no rights of monitoring and control, yet who are responsible for virtually all
treatment services outside hospitals and for intial identification of
patients to be treated inside; (2) organisational divisions between
GP and specialist services, which, in turn, have led to irrational
divisions between hospital and community health services; (3)
health authority reliance on local government social services
departments for the basic support of patients unable to look after
themselves, many of whom have to be hospitalised in order to
receive this; (4) failure of the DHSS to make realistic facilities
(including financial support) available to families for home
nursing, quickly and realistically enough to make it economically
viable, when the alternative of institutional care would be
demonstrably cheaper and less incommodious for the family.

When Aneuran Bevan submitted to GP demands for continu-
ation of *per capita* payments for 'list' or 'panel' patients as a
condition of their involvement in NHS work (a condition he may
have felt obliged to accept in order to get his Bill through
Parliament), he laid the foundations for a dissemination of NHS
resources which, arguably, has ever since prevented health
authorities from planning in the most appropriate consumer
interests. This is agreed by a large minority of emerging GPs (and

some of earlier generations), who hold the view that they could work more effectively than at present by joining forces with nurses, paramedical and social workers based in health centres linked with district hospitals. This view is seldom articulated because even its most ardent proponents concede that they currently enjoy freedoms and opportunities for personal advancement and independent activity which, they fear, might not apply if they were accountable to health authorities. They do not, however, accept that health centre development and their health authority employment would interfere with opportunities for family doctoring – and, in particular, close and lasting doctor–patient relationships – a claim frequently made by GPs opposed to this. Indeed, they believe these could be enhanced through better patient treatment and care, made possible by their access to health authority resources now denied to them: that they would open up for GPs long yearned-for prospects of participation in the mainstream of hospital medicine.

As far as hospital medicine is concerned, many problems which stem from reliance on medical teams composed largely of doctors (many newly fledged) occupying short-stay posts might be resolved, given the presence of fully experienced doctors (as are most GPs) in permanent posts covering general hospital beds as well as external health centre activity.

Clearly, district health authorities require *some* organisational divisions to meet their wide-ranging commitments. I have concluded existing ones of hospitals/community to be out of keeping with modern diagnostic and treatment requirements on the one hand, health education and the prevention of illness on the other. Where then do I think dividing lines should be drawn?

Establishment of health centres as part of district hospital complexes would open the way for logical authority planning towards, in one direction, prevention, early diagnosis and treatment, and in the other, treatment and care (in hospital or at home) of patients with complex high level needs. This would require the establishment of two distinct health care divisions – (i) primary and (ii) secondary – each with direct access to resources traditionally held in hospitals: (i) for epidemiological, educational and other prevention-orientated activities; (ii) for, ultimately, the practice of total patient care. From thence it would be possible to proceed with organisational arrangements according to types of cases presented (for example, minor illness, maternity, child welfare), each service having its own expertise according to case requirements in terms of specialist need, nursing and basic and social support. This would open the way, not only for the development of domiciliary alternatives to general hospital admission, but also for progress in all other branches of health care.

Only a comparatively small percentage of patients is likely at a given time to require hospital levels and varieties of treatment and care. In the event of domiciliary provision parallel to that traditionally available in general hospitals, sensitive and wide-ranging preassessment is required to determine who these patients are; the nature of their needs; the extent to which these needs might be willingly and ably met from members of patients' own entourages; which should be met by health authorities; which by other statutory services; and which, in the form of additional comforts, might be met through the mobilisation of voluntary effort.

I have therefore concluded that domiciliary provision for these patients should be the responsibility of secondary not primary health care services. Nevertheless, since most medical and nursing domiciliary care skills traditionally rest with the latter, I have recognised a crucial need to draw from them the experience and expertise necessary to establish 'hospital at home' as an integrated service combining hospital and community facilities.

Since health authorities are not statutorily permitted to make secondary care provision outside their hospital divisions, they are currently faced with an inescapable dilemma. They *must* provide hospital beds for patients who neither desire nor essentially require admission, because they cannot afford to allocate high levels and wide varieties of staff and resources necessary for their domiciliary care, to community nursing divisions whose operations are largely determined by the use independently contracted GPs make of them. The pre-assessment of cases potentially suitable for secondary home care cannot be properly assured by these nursing divisions because GPs are largely free to decide for themselves the extent to which community nurses shall be drawn into the home care of the sick.

It is commonly held that much waste in the NHS stems from the fact that large numbers of patients consult their doctors over trivial problems they are capable of resolving for themselves. The medical profession is in large part to blame for this. It has undermined lay confidence in accepting personal responsibility in decision making over health matters by establishing for itself an aura of omnipotence in the subject. Furthermore, it has not lived up to expectations of it in the pursuit of preventive medicine through health education.

My findings suggest that opportunities for decision making by patients implicit in HAH proposals (which would come into play at the point of pre-assessment of cases referred for admission) would encourage the *minimum* necessary use of secondary level resources allocated for use outside hospitals. Release by health authorities of such resources for distribution solely through existing GP services would, however, encourage their *maximum* use, not necessarily in directions where they were most needed.

Given that patients and their families are fully acquainted with what, in the event of a home care option, HAH could and could not offer, fully informed by their doctors as to medical matters involved, and reassured by the latter that an option in favour of HAH would not influence quality and quantity of medical care provided, and that, in the event of it proving too great a strain on the family, the alternative of hospital admission would be provided, my findings suggest that family expectations of outside help in the presence of illness would be modest. Indeed, I have found that professionals tend to rate needs higher than necessary when resources are readily at hand to satisfy them.

I now turn to changes necessary to assure the adequate nursing and basic support of the dependent sick outside hospitals. These must include domestic and social elements referred to widely in the nursing profession as 'non-nursing' and for which nurses traditionally bear no formal responsibility.

In most cases families, where present, willingly and ably accept the brunt of responsibility for the home care of sick members. Outside help where required is usually available from community health and social services; but not always at levels and of varieties necessary to relieve families from threat of breakdown.

Whilst anxious to acknowledge individual endeavours of nurses and other caring personnel allocated to their cases, patients' relatives point to the stresses and anxieties of not being certain of the kinds of help with which they will be provided, on what days, at what times of the day and for how long; they also indicate the problems of not being able to refer to someone 'in charge' who will co-ordinate all the various services being provided, making sure that these meet with those for which they themselves bear responsibility.

Who should ensure the care and basic support of the sick necessary to enable effective medical treatment when caring relatives are not able to do so in part or in whole?

In hospitals, the answer is clear – the ward sister. Even where a particular 'item' required is not specific to nursing, the ward sister nonetheless must make sure it is provided, in level and in kind, according to each individual patient's minimum needs and according to medical prescription.

I have concluded in 'hospital at home' a need for 'nurse-managers' who would be allocated overall case responsibility for patients admitted to the scheme. Of course, work in a domiciliary environment requires certain professional and personal qualities different from those required of nurses in hospital; it makes demands different from, although potentially as onerous as (or more onerous than), those of some hospital work. But whereas, from the old days of the hospital matron (responsible for laundry, catering and domestic services as well as nursing) onwards, *total* patient care has been intrinsic to in-hospital provision, community nursing has always consisted of providing discrete 'items' – and only specifically nursing items at that. Small wonder then that so many patients have to be hospitalised largely to provide for their general care and basic support!

Study of nursing history reveals a dichotomy of professional interests. One side favours advancement as of priority in the direction of developing clinical techniques. The other (apart from carrying out prescribed treatments) 'looking after' the patient, without firm lower limits as to kinds of duties involved. Of course, this is a broad generalisation. All nurses will assure us that their duties are primarily to ensure the patient's well-being regardless of what this involves. But community nurses are traditionally resistant to attempts to formalise their work, preferring to interpret need and sense of commitment from case to case.

As hospital procedures become increasingly sophisticated and more is required of nurses in the direction of technological and scientific expertise, hospital nursing has been rationalised, requiring, for example, specialist expertise in theatre, intensive care and other special units. Hence, while ward sisters have management responsibilities in the general care of large numbers of patients, other high grade nurses act more as clinical assistants, their responsibilities to patients being related only to small numbers during the time that specific procedures are taking place.

As district nurses are responsible for providing only 'items' of patient care, their daily rounds are usually of a size and content which prevents their acceptance of overall responsibility for any individual case. So where is the species of nurse to be found who could fulfil the case-management function for the home-bound dependent sick whose families cannot themselves adequately fulfil this?

The concept of 'hospital at home' implies a need for a new category of nurses in the NHS, orientated towards total patient care in domiciliary settings; that the nursing profession should reconsider its attitude to elements of care traditionally referred to as 'non-nursing'. If it is accepted that patients requiring high levels and wide varieties of care do not invariably require hospital admission, but that, at the same time, their families may not be able to 'manage' their cases, it is surely to the nursing profession that we must look for satisfactory solutions to alternatives of domiciliary care.

In 1970 the French Government accepted in principle that hospital treatment might, subject to the agreement of the patient's doctor, be continued in the patient's home (see page 73). This enabled hospital authorities to develop extramural care, subject to very stringent conditions, so that patients requiring up to total care might be provided for through integrated authority/family support. French *hospitalisation à domicile* services, established by many regional hospital authorities by virtue of the provision, employ multi-disciplinary aides working under nursing management towards this end. Nurses delegated case-management responsibility are able to call upon hospital authority resources assessed necessary to enable these aides to fulfil their roles.

Publication of the French experience in the early 1970s led some district health authorities in the UK to employ such aides

(HAH Peterborough called them 'patients' aides' to stress that they were not to be regarded as uniquely nursing auxiliaries). Inevitably, since, in contrast to the situation in France, there is no NHS provision in the UK for domiciliary patient support *not* of a nursing kind, the nature and extent of patient' aides' duties in the direction of 'non-nursing' elements of their work has never been formally established, any more than has that of the nurses delegated responsibility for the supervision and management of these aides. Of course (we hope) nurse and aide will apply such dedication and goodwill to each patient case that, in practice, both will do whatever requires to be done. But this does not provide UK health authorities with powers of monitoring and control over home care personnel and resources considered essential by French hospital authorities for the assurance of *guaranteed* minimum economic, effective and humane operation.

Although nursing management must be the lynchpin of comprehensive planning for the domiciliary care of the dependent sick, there must at the same time be provision for the intervention of paramedical and social workers: paramedical workers to oversee medically prescribed rehabilitation including (particularly in the case of the terminally ill) diversion and relief from pain; social workers for the fulfilment of functions which cannot be properly ascribed to nursing or general administration. Relations between paramedical workers and nurses can best be described by returning to the ward sister analogy: the doctor prescribes; the nurse is responsible for co-ordinating paramedical contributions with other elements of the patient's treatment and care. The functions of social workers must include elements additional upon those which are medically prescribed: social pre-assessment of cases referred for domiciliary comprehensive care; on-going social support of patients admitted; arrangements for satisfactory discharge arrangements when the patient no longer requires the presence of the service. The French have been able to make highly satisfactory arrangements for requisite social worker input into their *hospitalisation à domicile* schemes. But then, their hospital authorities employ their own social workers while health authorities in the UK do not.

The *National Health Service Reorganisation Act 1973* (Clause 18(4)(a)) did untold harm to the future of social medicine when it described medical social workers as being wholly or mainly employed in functions described under the Local Government Social Services Act of 1970. Thereafter their specialist training and qualification was abandoned: health authorities were required to call upon local authority social services departments for the social work support which they felt they needed; the latter were required to provide it in so far as they thought it feasible and necessary (*NHS Reorganisation Act 1973*, Clause 12(2)). This legislation has reflected particularly badly on the home-bound sick and disabled because their interests are not the overall responsibility of any particular statutory authority, as is the case during their presence in hospitals and other residential institutions.

The demise of medical social work in the NHS has left community nurses with onerous (if only moral) responsibilities to watch over the social interests of the cases they attend. Accordingly these have been incorporated in job descriptions, drawn up in consultation with them by senior nursing administrators. The extent to which these are met in practice is obscure, but it must be limited because, regardless of individual commitment, the machinery whereby nurses might gain even minimum satisfactory services for patients in their charge is lacking.

Health and social services professionals on one side, chronically disabled persons (who may nevertheless not be ill) on the other, may question the discretion of an approach to home care which makes firm distinctions between persons undergoing medical treatment and others, perhaps equally disadvantaged, who are not. This question taxed me when I first studied overseas home care schemes described in chapters 4 and 5. I hope that after reading this book my critics will agree with my conclusions that, in terms of organisation, these distinctions are fundamental to proper health and social services planning. Existing confusion is responsible for much unnecessary public suffering which stems from the incapacity of, respectively, treatment and non-treatment services to define, precisely, the disadvantaged population groups for which they are basically responsible. Theoretically, broad agreement exists between respective services about kinds of *institutional* care which should be provided for respective groups. (Although, in practice, 'rule of thumb' methods of allocation may be applied.) Outside institutions, even theoretical distinctions appear to be lacking.

Despite the fact that my proposals for 'hospital at home' would establish a dividing line between, on the one side, treatment and care facilities based on hospitals and, on the other, health and social services facilities which rely on external medical intervention as and when the need is indicated in an individual case, I believe they would ultimately enhance provision on both sides. This is because the establishment of such a dividing line would oblige health and social services authorities to face up to commitments they are currently able to evade by 'buck-passing'.

I also believe that the existence of extramural hospital services of the kind described in this book would oblige the medical profession to come to terms with the fact that what happens to health and social services consumers *not* of medical interest is of crucial significance to what happens to those who *are*.

Just as hospital beds are now frequently blocked by patients who have no medical need of them, HAH 'beds' would rapidly suffer the same fate if the doctors accepting clinical responsibility for the patients admitted to them manifested no interest beyond that of a clinical kind. Only, in the case of HAH, availability of hospital beds would not be a decisive factor in determining numbers of cases undertaken. Discharge from HAH would not, as is presently the case in hospitals, absolve the doctor holding clinical charge of a case from on-going responsibility, because that doctor would be the patient's GP.

I hope readers of this book have not gained the impression that my proposals cut across principles of family doctoring. Nothing could be further from their intentions. I hope I have succeeded in convincing readers that, without the organisational capacity to incorporate multi-disciplinary skills, and wide varieties and high levels of resources, it cannot in reality live up to these principles.

No government or authority is likely to favour health innovations likely to prove more costly than present health care provisions. To date there has been no experiment in the NHS capable of proving potential economies on general hospital provision, given the presence of parallel domiciliary provision. This is because NHS legislation, structure and organisation do not provide for it. Nevertheless, I am convinced that certain overseas health systems far more cost-conscious than our own would not have countenanced widespread experiment, followed by permanent adoption of schemes offering certain patients options between hospital admission and 'hospital at home' (or HAH-type) schemes, had the latter not proved demonstrably cheaper to operate and susceptible to effective monitoring and control.

Potential economy of such schemes to health authorities is, however, only half of the story. What of the cost of home care alternatives to hospital admission for patients and their families?

We recall that overseas schemes described insist that, given medical requirements of prior general hospital admission and GP willingness to accept clinical responsibility, rights of options in favour of domiciliary alternatives rest uniquely with patients and their caring relatives. This element of consumer choice enables the latter to reach decisions which have taken family cost factors into account. Overseas home care schemes mentioned above rest on the principle that services provided shall cost the patient no more than they would if provided in hospital. In countries like France, where hospital admission charges for most cases likely to be suitable for a domiciliary home care parallel are reimbursable at 100 per cent, this acknowledges in principle that patients requiring comprehensive treatment and care should receive it free of charge, even though this might be achieved through insurance regulations rather than those of nationalised health care. The extent to which patients opt for this parallel, despite the fact that it might involve additional family expenditure on items traditionally known in hospitals as 'hotel' costs, is a measure of their esteem for it.

Clearly, proposals put forward in this book require closer and more critical examination than I personally have been able to carry out in the limited space and with the limited resources available to me. My conviction as to the intrinsic potential value of 'hospital at home' stems partly from my experience during many years of medical social work in London, seeking in vain for satisfactory alternatives to hospital admissions, unwanted by patients and agreed unnecessary by patients' doctors, partly from first-hand experience of *hospitalisation à domicile* schemes operated by French hospital authorities, and partly from first-hand experience of the Peterborough experiment.

Apart from *hospital at home* potential to provide alternative parallels to hospital admission, one factor alone is sufficient to merit its introduction to the NHS. That is its concept of an organisation capable of integrating contributions of specialists and GPs, hospital and community services, towards patterns of patient care which give priority to the interests of the patient – a concept which the NHS, both in its original form and under subsequent reorganisations, has so far significantly failed to demonstrate.

It now rests with health politicians, professionals and administrators, and patients' representatives to determine future opportunities for those of us needing hospital level and type care to be provided with it in the security and comfort of our own homes.

Appendix A: Some cost findings on the home care of the sick – a reference list

Butler, J. R., and Pearson, M., *Who Goes Home?* Occasional Papers on Social Administration No. 34, B. Bell & Sons, London, 1970.

Colt, A. M., *et al.*, 'Home health care is good economics', *Nursing Outlook*, October 1977, 632–6.

Creese, A. L., and Fielden, R., 'Hospital or home care for the severely disabled: a cost comparison', *British Journal of Social and Preventive Medicine*, 1977, **31**, 116–21.

Doherty, N., and Hicks, B., 'Cost-effectiveness analysis and alternative health care programs for the elderly. *Health Services Research*, 1977, **12**(2), 190–203.

Donaldson, S. N., *et al.*, 'Demand for patient care', *British Medical Journal*, 1977, *ii*, 799–802.

Echeverri, O., *et al.*, 'Postoperative care: in hospital or at home?' *International Journal of Health Services*, 1972, **2**(1), 101–10.

Gerson, L. W., and Berry, A. F. E., 'Psycho-social effects of home care: results of a randomised controlled trial', *International Journal of Epidemiology*, 1976, **5**(2), 159–65.

Gerson, L. W., and Collins, J. F., 'A randomised controlled trial of home care: clinical outcome for five surgical procedures', *The Canadian Journal of Surgery*, November 1976, 519–523.

Gibbins, F. H., *et al.*, 'Augmented home nursing as an alternative to hospital care for chronic elderly invalids', *British Medical Journal*, 1982, **284**, 330–3.

Hunt, T. E., *et al.*, 'One third of a million days of care at home, 1959–1975', *Canadian Medical Association Journal*, 1977, **116**(12), 1351–5.

Lewis, D., and Mackey, M., 'Home care program cuts dollars and days', *Canadian Hospital*, 1973, **50**(5), 37–40.

Mackintosh, J. M., *et al.*, 'An examination of the need for hospital admission', *The Lancet*, 1961, *i*, 815–8.

Opit, L. J., 'Domiciliary care for the elderly sick – economy or neglect?' *British Medical Journal*, 1977, *i*, 30–3.

Pasker, P., and Ashley, J. S. A., 'Inter-relationship of different sectors of the total health and social services system', *Community Medicine*, 12 November 1971, 271–6.

Rickard, J. H., 'The costs of domiciliary nursing care', *Journal of the Royal College of General Practitioners*, 1974, **24**, 839–45.

Seidl, F. W., *et al.*, 'Is home care less expensive?' *Health and Social Work*, 1977, **2**(2), 5–19.

Warner, J. D., and Kolff, W. U., 'Cost of home dialysis versus institutional dialysis, *Journal of Dialysis*, 1976, **1**(1), 67–73.

Widmer, G., *et al.*, 'Home health care: services and cost', *Nursing Outlook*, August 1978, 488–93.

Wolcott, L. E., *et al.*, 'Home care vs. institutional rehabilitation of stroke: a comparative study', *Missouri Medicine*, 1966, **63**(9), 722–4.

Relative Costs of Home Care and Nursing Home and Hospital Care in Australia, Monograph Series No. 10, Commonwealth Department of Health, Canberra, 1979.

Appendix B: Selected book list

Abel-Smith, B., *The Hospitals, 1800–1948*, Heinemann, London, 1964.
Abel-Smith, B., *History of the Nursing Profession*, Heinemann, London, 1960.
Balint, E., and Norell, J. S., *Six Minutes for the Patient*, Tavistock, London, 1973, and Social Science Paperbacks, London, 1976.
Balint, M., *The Doctor, His Patient and the Illness*, Pitman, London, 1964.
Bevan, A., *In Place of Fear*, MacGibbon and Kee, London, 1961.
Bowling, A., *Delegation in General Practice*, Tavistock, London, 1981.
Brown, R. G. S., *The Changing National Health Service*, Routledge and Kegan Paul, London, 1973.
Bullough, V. L., and Bullough, B., *The Care of the Sick*, Croom Helm, London, 1979.
Byrne, P. S., and Long, B. E., *Doctors Talking to Patients*, HMSO, London, 1976.
Butler, J., *Family Doctors and Public Policy*, Routledge and Kegan Paul, London, 1973.
Cartwright, A., *Human Relations and Hospital Care*, Routledge and Kegan Paul, London, 1964.
Cartwright, A., *Patients and Their Doctors*, Routledge and Kegan Paul, London, 1967.
Cartwright, A., *Patients and Their Doctors in 1977*, Royal College of General Practitioners, London, 1982.
Cartwright, A., and Anderson, R., *General Practice Revisited*, Tavistock, London, 1981.
Donnison, J., *Midwives and Medical Men*, Schocken Books, New York, 1977.
Doyal, L., *The Political Economy of Health*, Pluto Press, 1979.
Dunnel, K., and Cartwright, A., *Medicine Takers, Prescribers and Hoarders*, Routledge and Kegan Paul, London, 1972.
Ehrenreich, B., and English, D., *Witches, Midwives and Nurses: A History of Women Healers*, Writers and Readers Publishing Cooperative, London, 1976.
Goldman, L., *Angry Young Doctor*, Hamish Hamilton, London, 1957.

Hodson, M., *Doctors and Patients*, Hodder and Stoughton, London, 1967.

Honigsbaum, F., *The Division in British Medicine*, Kogan Page, London, 1979.

Iliffe, S., *The NHS: A Picture of Health*, Lawrence and Wishart, London, 1983.

Illich, I., *Medical Nemesis*, Calder and Boyars, London, 1975; revised edition entitled *Limits in Medicine*, 1976.

Illich, I., *The Disabling Professions: Ideas in Progress*, Marion Boyars, London, 1977.

Jaques, E., *Health Services*, Heinemann Educational, London, 1978.

Jefferys, M., and Sachs, H., *Re-thinking General Practice*, Tavistock, London, 1983.

Levitt, R., *The Reorganised National Health Service*, Croom Helm, London, 1976.

Melville, A., and Johnson, C., *Cured to Death*, Secker and Warburg, London, 1982.

Perry, N., and Perry, J., *The Rise of the Medical Profession*, Croom Helm, London, 1976.

Pollack, K., *The Healers*, Nelson, London, 1968.

Stewart, M. C., *My Brother's Keeper*, Health Horizons, London, 1968.

Stoddard, S., *The Hospice Movement*, Jonathan Cape, London, 1979.

Townsend, P., and Davidson, N., *The Black Report*, Penguin Books, Harmondsworth, 1982.

Tudor Hart, J., *The National Health Service in England and Wales: A Marxist Perspective*, Marxists in Medicine, London, 1976.

Webb, S., and Webb, B., *English Poor Law Policy*, Longman, London, 1910.

Webb, S., and Webb, B., *English Poor Law Policy: Part II*, Longman, London, 1929.

Webb, S., and Webb, B., *The State and the Doctor*, Longman, London, 1910.

Widgery, D., *Health In Danger*, Macmillan, London, 1979.

Willcocks, A. J., *The Creation of the National Health Service*, Routledge and Kegan Paul, London, 1967.

Woodward, J., *To Do the Sick No Harm*, Routledge and Kegan Paul, London, 1974.

Zorza, R., and Zorza, V., *A Way to Die: Living to the End*, André Deutsch, London, 1980.

Appendix C: Official publications

Interim Report on the Future Provision of Medical and Allied Services (Chairman: Lord Dawson), HMSO, London, 1920.

Social Insurance and Allied Services: Report by Sir William Beveridge, Cmnd 6404, HMSO, London, 1942.

A National Health Service, HMSO, London, 1944.

The National Health Service Act 1946, HMSO, London, 1946.

Report of the Committee on Local Authority and Allied Personal Social Services (Chairman: F. Seebohm), Cmnd 3703, HMSO, London, 1968.

The National Health Service Reorganisation Act 1973, HMSO, London, 1973.

The Organisation of the In-patient's Day: Report of a Committee of the Central Health Services Council (Chairman: Sir John Hanbury), HMSO, London, 1976.

Byrne, P. S., and Long, B. E., *Doctors Talking to Patients*, HMSO, London, 1976.

Report of the Royal Commission on the National Health Service (Chairman: Sir Alec Merrison), HMSO, London, 1979.

Inequalities in Health: Report of a Research Working Group (Chairman: Sir Douglas Black), DHSS, London, 1982; see also Townsend, P., and Davidson, N., *The Black Report*, Penguin Books, Harmondsworth, 1982.

Index